Dr Peter O'Connor, PhD, BA, MAPsS,
is a psychologist who conducts a private adult
psychotherapy practice in Melbourne, Australia. He
has a special professional interest in dreams and as
part of his practice conducts weekly dream analysis
groups. He is also the author of several previous
books: *Mirror on Marriage* (1973), *Understanding the
Mid-Life Crisis* (1982), *Dreams and the Search for Meaning*
(1986), *Understanding Jung* (1985), *The Inner Man*
(1993). His next book, *Beyond the Mist*, will be
published in 2001.

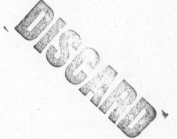

PETER A. O'CONNOR

FACING
THE
FIFTIES

*from denial
to reflection*

ALLEN & UNWIN

First published in 2000

Allen & Unwin
9 Atchison Street
St Leonards NSW 2065
Australia
Phone: (61 2) 8425 0100
Fax: (61 2) 9906 2218
Email: frontdesk@allen-unwin.com.au
Web: http://www.allenandunwin.com

National Library of Australia
Cataloguing-in-Publication entry:

O'Connor, Peter A., 1942 –.
Facing the fifties: from denial to reflection.

ISBN 1 86508 384 4.

1. Aging – Psychological aspects. 2. Aged – Attitudes.
I. Title.

305.26

Cover photograph by Jim Brandenburg:
Australian Picture Library/Minden Pictures
Cover and text design by Sandra Nobes
Index by Shirley Johnston
Set in 12 pt Weiss by Midland Typesetters
Printed by Australian Print Group

10 9 8 7 6 5 4 3 2

Contents

to Margaret

Acknowledgments

This book is ostensibly the work of one person, but in truth it owes its existence to many. First, I would like to acknowledge my debt to the individuals who so generously and openly gave of their time to be interviewed for the project. Their names and details have been deliberately altered in the text in order to protect their anonymity, but the value of their contributions is openly acknowledged; without them, this book would not have been possible. Second, I thank my colleagues and friends who recommended subjects to be interviewed: Felix Carrady, Kaalii Cargill, Brian Clark, Michelle de Jong, Susanne Romanin, Donna Ward and Damian West. To the members of my dream groups, I record a special thanks for stimulating my interest in the subject and for the ongoing education they have given me.

On a more personal note, I need to thank Andrew, Veronica and Michelle of Food For All Seasons in Warrandyte. Their delightful ambience and excellent coffee provided a much-needed escape. Glennys Lawton's and Brian Clark's friendship and kindness was invaluable, particularly their practical help at a critical time of the writing. Christine Bright deserves a special thank-you because she sensitively and intelligently transferred the material from paper to computer in a way that was seamless.

Finally, to my wife Margaret I acknowledge my deepest gratitude. Not only has she been a great friend and support but also a sensitive and thoughtful sounding-board and critic. Her editing of the early draft substantially improved the manuscript and made it eminently more readable.

Peter O'Connor
Melbourne, 2000

Preface

It is twenty years since I wrote *Understanding the Mid-Life Crisis*. The cohort that I was writing about then are now all in their mid- to late fifties, a very different stage in life from the mid-thirties. This book emerges out of a slowly maturing reflection on what being in the fifties is like and how it reflects, contrasts with, or continues the crises of mid-life.

These vaguely formed thoughts were given extra impetus through my professional work with groups of individuals wishing to explore their dream life. These are long-term groups, and over the past year or two an increasing number of members have moved into their fifties. It became readily apparent that this transition, engineered by our biological clocks, did not go unnoticed at the unconscious level, regardless of whether a person was focussing on it consciously or not. Dreams about ageing, conflict over appearances, sexual attractiveness, regrets about youth, anxieties about physical deterioration and finally acute anxiety about death all began to appear in the groups. Sometimes individuals would dream of aged or dead parents, and the ensuing discussion would open up the vexed area of old age and ageing. Other dreams depicted figures from the past, who served to remind the dreamer of lost opportunities and foregone choices; and feelings of envy often accompanied these images. Dreams of certain articles of clothing would remind the dreamer of lost youth and freedom. Clothes and styles from the 1960s symbolise for most dreamers in their fifties a time of vibrancy, carefreeness and endless opportunity.

These dreams and the many rich discussions of them that ensued awakened in me a desire to explore the experience of being in the fifties. This desire had already been stirred by my own experience of turning fifty. The process of writing affords me an opportunity for self-exploration and reflection, a process I first started as a late teenager as I struggled with the tumult of adolescence and renewed in mid-life as I was confronted with questions of identity and work. So naturally when I moved into my fifties and began to experience new and unknown feelings and images, my thoughts turned to writing. The central and dominant theme of the images that emerged over this period was that of my own death, and the grief associated with the loss of youth and all that went with it. As the fifties progressed, these feelings and images began to give way to a growing sense that dying with a measure of conscious awareness was the next developmental task.

This did not feel morbid, and it certainly did not imply that I ought to get on with the task of dying immediately. Rather what these thoughts did achieve was to establish a renewed sense of meaning where in the immediately preceding years there had been a void. This meaning was to hold in consciousness the thought of one's own mortality as a background against which to live and sort out priorities and values. Dreams have always been a valuable source of reflection throughout both my personal and professional life, and the experience of the fifties proved no exception. My dreams were replete with images of decay and renewal, themes that were constantly repeated in my discussions with people in their fifties. As at mid-life, through these discussions and the dream groups, I discovered that I was not alone; the tyranny of privacy had once again been overcome. I hope this book serves the same purpose for its readers, since in the act of acknowledging our common struggles and dilemmas we enhance our compassion and humanity.

As I had done in exploring the experience of mid-life, I chose to start with people's own accounts of this time in their lives, in the form of an unstructured interview with sixty people, both men and women. These were people I had asked to participate, or people who had heard on the grapevine about the project. The interviews were designed not so much to gather facts as to provide a space in which the feeling experience of being in one's fifties could be shared and explored. My clear goal was to explore the feelings and themes involved in being between fifty and sixty years of age, but I did not start out with any set questions. I collected, and the interviewees often re-collected, their stories, their plots, their *mythos*, and each was rich and complex.

Whilst the research work I did on mid-life seemed complex, it finally yielded a fairly uniform and predictable set of themes and struggles. The transition into our fifties is neither well-defined nor predictable: indeed its most distinguishing feature is variability, and there were times during the interviews when I felt that no identifiable pattern actually existed. Being in one's fifties does seem to bring with it a desire to do things one's own way, and this in itself accounts in part for the range of experiences. Nevertheless, within this remarkable variability some persistent themes did emerge and they form the basis of this book. I do not wish to suggest that what is discussed in this book is applicable to *all* people in their fifties. Clearly, the sample was biased. There was no attempt on my part to conform to the sampling dictums of social science. However, I can say in what manner the group was biased: they were educated, middle-class, and generally well-off and successful. Biased maybe, but nevertheless they do represent a large number of people, people who are experiencing the uncertainty of being in their fifties and seeking to reflect on and to bring some measure of conscious awareness to the experience.

One of the operating deceptions of "social science"

research is that so-called scientific methodology renders the studies reliable. Whilst methodology is important, more often than not a rigid obsession with pure methodology is at the expense of content, and thus one often finishes up with a reliable piece of trivia, with the *only* significance being a statistical one. No doubt my methods, (or as some will perceive it, the lack of them) will again attract the ire of academically oriented psychologists, as happened when my work on mid-life came out. At that time it was criticised for being anecdotal or purely subjective. Yet the book has been continuously in print for nineteen years, which suggests that the subject is of intense interest and that the use of story and anecdotal evidence is seen by many as a valid source of understanding. I hold the view that to understand human nature, we need stories, metaphors and images, not laboratories, questionnaires and statistics. Poets and novelists articulate and give image to universal feeling issues and dilemmas, and they are often well ahead of psychology in their understanding of human nature. There is no notion on my part that this is a definitive or objective account of ageing through the fifties. I will leave that fantasy to academics! I have simply attempted to weave together some consistent strands that appeared throughout the interviews and to place these strands in some sort of order that assists reflection.

As the interviews proceeded I began to see that while some themes were common across the decade, the early fifties were more characterised by talk of loss and separation from youth and the grief associated with this, and people in their middle fifties made far more references to uncertainty and ambiguity than those in their early or late fifties. In time I came to appreciate that the separation, initiation and return paradigm of a rite of passage expressed the pattern of differences that I had observed. Separation is basic to all change and of necessity it entails giving something up, which in turn can evoke a deep and abiding sense of grief. Mourning is a natural psychological healing process not only for the death of someone we were attached to, but also for the loss of anything that was important to us and gave us some sense of meaning. Within the psychoanalytic tradition, the process of successful mourning is considered to be critical for the development of symbolic and imaginative thought, which allows one to develop an inner-directed life and leads to the next stage of initiation. This second stage, the middle fifties, is characterised by ambiguity and uncertainty and could best be described as a liminal, betwixt and between state. But it is also the space in which change occurs, as in the very fluidity of a liminal space one is open to the beginnings of renewal. It is thus the phase in which we can be initiated into a different sense of ourselves to replace those aspects that have been lost and grieved for. From a psychoanalytic point of view, tolerance of ambiguity within ourselves is the outcome of a reparation process whereby we have moved towards acknowledging and accepting our own destructiveness, a process stimulated by awareness of one's inevitable death. The corollary of this acceptance is greater integration and a renewed sense of self, and these constitute the "return" phase of the paradigm. Thus the rite of passage model of separation, initiation and return, when combined with psychoanalytical knowledge of mourning and reparation, facilitates an understanding of what it means to be in one's fifties.

1

Ageing or Old?

The phenomenon of the mid-life crisis which I first wrote about in 1979 is now well entrenched in social consciousness. Although there is an increasing tendency to use it as a causal explanation these days for a whole range of behaviours that may or may not be attributable to the mid-life transition, there is also a growing, notably American, tendency to extend the age during which one considers mid-life to occur to include people within the fifty-year-old bracket. This expansion of the age range of mid-life perhaps reflects the persistence and strength of the wish not to be old (we're not old, we're just in the midst of a mid-life crisis). The fact is that if we see fifty as mid-life, then we're expecting to live to a hundred! Traditionally, mid-life is considered to be the period between thirty-five and forty-five years of age, and it represents the stage of transition into middle adulthood.

As with all transitions, the "mid-life" period signifies change, change that is biologically driven and occurring continuously but which becomes apparent during a stage one can identify or name. Transitions involve a reappraisal of our present situations and structure, the exploring of new possibilities for oneself in the world which are more congruent with our emerging age and the working towards these possibilities through the process of making choices and foregoing old structures. The word "crisis" itself is derived from the Greek word *krisis*, meaning to sift. Therefore, transitional crises are periods of sifting. But that makes it sound as if it is an even and straightforward, logical process, whereas the experience of any transition is not like that at all. Central to all developmental stages is a mixture of anxiety and loss, of hope and despair, of anger and sadness. In short, every transition introduces, by necessity, the experience of mourning and grief, since all transitions inevitably evoke loss as a prelude to renewal and change.

Mid-life is but one of life's transitions, since clearly developmental stages occur throughout the life cycle. Infancy is followed by early childhood, ending at five to six years of age with the transition to school and the outside world and the necessary loss of the familiar home environment. A period of steady growth through latency is ended abruptly by the biological turbulence of puberty and emergence into adolescence, literally the stage of entering or moving into adulthood, with its socially identified and sanctioned emergence at eighteen and again at twenty-one. The period of young adulthood, involving many important tasks of relationship, marriage, children and work, along with a developing sense of individual identity, extends until the mid-life period, around thirty-five to forty-five. This period is typified by what has come to be known as "the mid-life crisis" and the moving into middle adulthood. One could consider the period of middle or mature adult-hood to extend for approximately ten to fifteen years from 50 – 65 with late adulthood beginning somewhere in the sixties. Beyond the age of seventy-five one can, I think, with some validity, begin to speak of old age. But from fifty that leaves approximately twenty to twenty-five years of middle and late adult life to be lived before one could be regarded as old.

What I found in researching for this book was that psychology and sociology have concentrated almost exclusively on old age per se. The burgeoning field of gerontology attests to this. The ample references on ageing, upon closer inspection, focused mainly on geri-atric themes of aged care and housing, for example—it is as if the content of gerontological studies reflects an undifferentiated anxiety among middle-aged academics concerning their own fears about getting old. I am not for one moment suggesting that gerontology is not a most valid and worthwhile area of concern; but I do want to invite some reflection as to what might lie behind this preoccupation with age rather than ageing. One way to defend against anxiety about getting old is to project it forward, distance it in time; then one can put one's efforts into issues concerning that seemingly "other" group of people, separate from oneself, that we can regard as the elderly. Here then is a fundamental split between the inevitable biological process of getting old, and the state of actually being elderly. Shelves and shelves of university libraries are devoted to studies on the aged, and yet there remains a deafening silence about the period between the late forties and the mid-sixties.

Is it that we all just get on with living an undisturbed life during this period and then one day we wake up and say to ourselves, "Now I am old"? This is what the bulk of current research would suggest—that is, that there is a future state called old age and via projection we can distance ourselves from the frail, sick and old people in need of care. What makes ageing such a difficult and complex experience is that we do not discriminate between ageing and death, between ageing and dependence, between ageing and the frailty of old age itself. In short we have turned a process into a fixed state, so ageing becomes old. Thus we have a poorly developed awareness of the process of ageing and have displaced our anxieties and fears out, into the future, onto another group of people we can distance ourselves from and call old. One can only wonder what the effects of these projections have been, and indeed still are, on the policies and programs developed to care for old people, since images of decrepitude seem to lie behind them.

Death is the inevitable outcome of life, but ageing is a stage or phase of life, not an outcome. This failure to differentiate between ageing and age indicates a regression to concrete literal thinking. This kind of literal, concrete thinking is invariably the sign of an underlying anxiety, and it suggests a failure to be aware of the feelings that may lie behind, or beneath the concretisation. Such a lack of awareness results in poor differentiation of the process of ageing, or indeed any experience, and the end result is a simplistic, stereotyped perception that denies ambiguity and complexity. Thus age comes to equal frailty, sickness and death, not also wisdom, freedom and an opportunity for continuing development.

Psychoanalysis and its derivatives, undoubtedly the major influence on our notions of psychological development, have also failed to explore and articulate the process of ageing. If gerontology mounts an institutionalised defence against age by putting it forward in the future, psychoanalysis has defended against the angst of ageing by going backwards to early childhood. With few exceptions, notably the pioneering work of the psychoanalyst Erik Erikson, and latterly the contributions of Peter Hildebrand of London and David Guttman, Robert Nemiroff and Calvin Colarusso in the United States, psychoanalysis has systematically ignored the process of ageing. Perhaps it has been subtly but powerfully influenced by the thoughts of its originator, Sigmund Freud. In 1904 he said,

If the patient's age is in the neighbourhood of their fifties, the conditions for psychoanalysis become unfavourable. The mass of psychic material is then no longer manageable; the time required for recovery is too long, and the ability to undo psychical processes begins to grow weaker.[1]

In another place (speaking of psychotherapy), he adds, "Near or above the age of fifty, the elasticity of the mental processes on which treatment depends is as a rule lacking—old people are no longer educable".[2]

These views of Freud's are both astonishing and sad. Astonishing insofar as he himself was in his late forties when he wrote this, and equally astonishing insofar as he continued to write and produce many major works well after the time he turned fifty. For example, Freud wrote his scholarly *Totem and Taboo* at fifty-seven, the classic work *Inhibition, Symptoms and Anxiety* at seventy and *Moses and Monotheism* at the ripe age of seventy-eight! What is sad is that these thoughts of Freud's, which are clearly inconsistent with his own life, have continued to influence, and in part shape, the practice, training and theories of psychoanalysis. For example, it is doubtful if anyone over forty could commence training as a psychoanalyst and it is certainly impossible for anyone over fifty. It would seem that Freud, in placing sexuality at the centre of his theory, may have assumed that the diminution and slowing down of sexuality in the fifties and beyond implied a similar slowing-down of the

mental faculties. As Peter Hildebrand in his fine book
Beyond Mid-Life Crisis asserts, psychoanalysts

> have far too uncritically accepted a hypothesis of contin-
> uous and physical intellectual development with a rising
> curve of growth from birth to adulthood, a long refrac-
> tory period and then a terminal stage of psychic deficit
> and social withdrawal preliminary to dying and death
> itself.[3]

The classical theory of psychoanalysis has a
tendency to reduce all explanations back to infancy and
early childhood experiences. While there can be absolutely no doubt that these are formative, they shape
rather than completely determine one's adult life. To
fail to hold this more dynamic view of interaction
between childhood and adult experiences and the environment, an interaction which continually adds to and
alters our psychic life, leads to a denial of the anxieties
involved in the present dilemmas of ageing. So the
danger is that within the world of classical psychoanalysis the very real losses and depression that come
with getting old are explained away by returning to the
earlier experience of childhood. Once again one can
see a displacement of the anxiety, this time not forward,
but backward. I don't suggest for one moment that the
past and the future have no effect on the present, but
to resort to one or other perspective as an exclusive
explanation is to deny recognition of current experience

—specifically the developmental phase that we might call ageing. The real value of the past is that it can be of considerable importance in throwing light on the present, just as thoughts and hopes about the future can reveal issues in the present.

There can be little doubt that the way an individual deals with the anxieties and challenges of any one developmental period will influence his or her capacity to deal with the next one. And whilst each stage of development has its own specific issues, it will also be affected by the experiences of similar issues and struggles from earlier periods. Even though adolescence has some unique aspects, specifically pubescence changes to the body, it is not uninfluenced by earlier childhood, particularly the sexual identity issues of the Oedipal phase, around five to six years of age. Mid-life likewise presents some uniquely specific issues of identity, but it is particularly shaped by the patterns and choices of adolescence and cannot be understood separately from this period. The approach taken throughout this book, therefore, is broadly speaking a psychodynamic one. I aim to explore the actual experience of being in a specific stage of one's life—the fifties—when certain issues and themes are faced for the first time, at least the first time consciously. I also intend, where appropriate, to make links between this phase and other phases of psychological development.

1 Sigmund Freud (1904), "Freud's Psycho-Analytic Procedure",
   Standard Edition vol. 7, Hogarth Press, London, 1953, pp. 249–56.
2 Sigmund Freud (1905), "On psychotherapy", op. cit., pp. 257–70.
3 Peter Hildebrand, *Beyond Mid-Life Crisis: A Psychodynamic Approach to
   Ageing*, Sheldon Press, London, 1995, p. 3.

2

The Life and Death Forces: Eros and Thanatos

As was mentioned earlier, despite considerable variation in people's responses to turning fifty, the one
consistent pattern was the experience of loss. It seems
it is no longer possible to deny the loss of youth,
although the denial appears to stay in place until
around the age of fifty-four to fifty-five. The early
fifties, and indeed the precise point of turning fifty,
are more characterised by feeling and identifying with
still being in the forties. So one hears most people
saying that they did not feel any different when they
turned fifty. This is partly denial, the initial mechanism used in grief for avoiding the pain of loss, but
is also a reflection of the fact that the experience of
the life cycle is a continuous process, not a series of
sudden discrete events. But by the mid-fifties, the
appearance of one's body tells the tale of being fifty-
something if nothing else does, and constellates a very
sad feeling of loss. Whilst some people focus on
specific issues such as the loss of physical and sexual

attractiveness, there are several other very real and substantial losses incurred with the ageing process. In one's mid-fifties these become somewhat painfully apparent, and often lead individuals to seek some form of psychotherapy.

1   There's a fear of diminution of one's sexual potency and attractiveness, and anxiety about the effect of this on present relationships and the possibility of future relationships.

2   In our modern world there's a very real pressure associated with the possible or actual loss of meaningful work, either through redundancy or voluntary retirement. This threatens the sense of identity and self-esteem, which can contribute to a feeling of worthlessness, despite the initial euphoria that many people feel on first giving up work.

3   The loss of children as they take leave of the family home to set up their own independent lives can expose deeper losses, particularly in the marital sphere. The children's departure often lifts the protective mask that has covered long-standing deficits in the marriage relationship which have been compensated for by the rewards of caring for children.

4   There is a loss of youthfulness, vigour and energy, and an anxiety that comes with the fearful anticipation of increasing frailty, sickness and increasing dependence on others for care.

5   The loss of mental acuity and short-term memory
    carries a threat of senility, even Alzheimer's disease.
6   The most powerful loss of all is a growing aware-
    ness of the loss of life itself—the realisation in one's
    fifties of the inevitability of one's own death.

On the surface this reads as a fairly depressing list, and one could readily appreciate anyone in their fifties pondering whether there was any point in going on, if all one could look forward to was loss. Of course loss is present in all transitions, but in each of them prior to the fifties transition one can also console oneself with there still being time ahead. In the fifties, that defensive strategy is difficult to maintain with much conviction. Such negativity has behind it a profound instinctual interplay pulling the strings of consciousness first in one direction and then in another, and sometimes even breaking a string, leaving us feeling totally moribund. What I am referring to is the archetypal interplay between Eros, the instinctual force that serves to connect, the life force, and Thanatos, the opposite force, the goal of which is disconnection and ultimately death.

It was Sigmund Freud in 1930, at the age of seventy-four, who so poignantly reflected upon this archetypal interaction when he said, "And now, I think, the meaning of the evolution of civilisation is no longer obscure to us. It must present the struggle between Eros and Death, between the instinct of life and the instinct of destruction".[1]

We can take the death instinct to be Thanatos, the ancient Greek mythological god of death who resided in Tartarus below Hades. Eros, is of course, the god of connection, who ought not be diminished into some bow-and-arrow-carrying cupid. On the contrary, in the Greek myths of creation, according to Hesiod, Eros is the primeval force that brings harmony to chaos and permits life to develop. This cosmic force of connection had little to do with the later versions of the god of love, although one can see how this would have naturally developed from his role as co-ordinator of the elements that constituted the universe. The reduction of Eros from a cosmic force of connection to an arrow-bearing cupid is continued in our present-day belittling of Eros as nothing more than sexual excitement and titillation. It seems as if there is always a desire in human beings to reduce the complex and the mysterious to a level of banal, concrete literality; perhaps it sells better at this level! But if Eros has been diminished in status then Thanatos, the cosmic force of disconnection and death, has been banished to the hinterland, out of sight and consciousness altogether, so that death becomes in our fantasy something that happens to others. Again Sigmund Freud had some succinct thoughts about this:

> We were prepared to maintain that death was the neces-
> sary outcome of life . . . In reality, however, we were
> accustomed to behave as if it were otherwise. We
> displayed an unmistakable tendency to "shelve" death, to

eliminate it from life. We tried to hush it up . . . No-one
believes in his own death . . . In the unconscious everyone is convinced of his own immortality.[2]

Yet these two powerful instinctual patterns in the
psyche find their origins in what one might call the
two biological imperatives, towards life and death. At
the level of the psyche these instincts are known as
Eros and Thanatos. These are the forces that act in
tandem from beginning to end of one's life, and indeed
could be considered as the energy of the life cycle
itself, without which it would not be. However it is
clear that they do not operate equally throughout the
life cycle: at certain points in time Eros will be in the
ascendancy and at others Thanatos. Yet in moments or
periods of transition we need both energies to make
possible the disconnection from one stage and the
connection to the next. To see Thanatos as only death
and destruction is to miss the point entirely—it is the
psychic force of disconnection, with death the final
disconnection. Our anxieties about death have limited
our conscious understanding of this fundamental
energy to simply seeing it as frightening and ultimately
destructive. Thanatos is no more just about death than
Eros is just about sex.

The relevance of this discussion to the perception of
loss that characterises the fifties is that loss activates
Thanatos and awakens thoughts of endings and death.
Just as we struggle so often not to split youth and age

and overlook the process of ageing, so also do we split life and death. In our anxiety about "the end", we rush headlong toward it and miss the scenery of the processes and endings that go on long before we reach our destination. We automatically equate "loss" with "end", and lurking behind our thoughts of "end" in our fifties lies the most fearful thought of all—*The End* that is death. So loss and the awakening of Thanatos are intrinsically connected and losses such as often occur in the fifties bring with the sadness and grief a profound sense of inevitable separation.

At this point Eros, the force of connection, is often very difficult to sustain in consciousness, and therefore we can sometimes feel there is no hope, no purpose, no point, no future and no sense of life. At moments of profound loss we are entirely in the grip of Thanatos who temporarily banishes Eros. Herein lies the profound angst of getting older, that moment when it really becomes apparent that youth has passed and age is truly commencing, that the body no longer lies!

At other stages in the life cycle, particularly adolescence and mid-life, the balance of the energies is more strongly in favour of the life force; Thanatos makes a brief appearance in consciousness at thirty-five or so, but often then recedes into the unconscious until the fifties. At the mid-life transition the desire for Eros to triumph over Thanatos and disconnection characteristically is reflected in sexual fantasies and sexual acting out.

Sexuality pursued for its own sake, in isolation from a feeling connection, as it often is in mid-life, is basically a means of protecting oneself from and denying the reality of one's death. The sexualisation of Eros is most common among men, where it serves this very purpose of overcoming separation anxiety and the dread of disconnection. So for many men the mid-life transition does not engender an increase in maturity and reflection, a shift from outer to inner, rather it shows a panic (or manic) flight away from reflection and acceptance of one's mortality into a pursuit of power, sex and status (a little like a middle-aged version of sex, drugs and rock'n'roll).

But reaching the fifties makes this solution more difficult, if not unsustainable, since now Thanatos hears the call, is beckoned into awareness by the subtle but inevitable deterioration of body, by the diminution of strength, sexual drive and physical well-being and attractiveness. By the mid-fifties a fundamental shift occurs, with time already lived outweighing time left to be lived before death. This shift is in my view the great initiator into a more fully realised life, since it brings with it the possibility, if we allow it, of altering our orientation from an outwardly directed one to an increasingly inward one. This is a profound psychological change, in which our centre of gravity moves away from the persona, the sense of being defined by outer sources, towards the self, the sense of being defined from within. This shift towards interiority brings with it a sense of relativity and continuity, and thereby alters one's sense of time and space. In short, if a successful shift is made to the centre of psychic gravity then one begins to experience oneself more directly rather than exclusively in terms of relationships with others. Whilst attachments can, and do, continue, separateness can be held alongside the attachment. However, the successful shift from outer to inner, from persona or false self to the self, involves a complex process of letting go, separating from preceding and fixed views of oneself and allowing oneself to go through a period of mourning and grief for those aspects that are now lost. This complex process of mourning forms the essential dynamic of the shift and is the focus of the next chapter.

The role of Thanatos in a transition is vital, since it is the very energy that creates the letting go, the separation. The goal of Thanatos is to disconnect, to deconstruct, but we rarely welcome its appearance on our psychic stage. Instead we hang on, and we rally Eros, the principle of connectedness, to our defence. But in many ways this is an inappropriate use of Eros and in some situations could be considered perverse, insofar as it perverts the course of the life cycle and creates the illusion of omnipotence—the belief that we can stop the movement of life itself. Cosmetic surgery, for example, while undoubtedly benefiting many people in the short term, is a process that will no doubt delay the outward appearance of ageing, but in the long run it cannot prevent the soul being aware of the inevitability of the process itself.

But just as using Eros to stay connected to the stage or phase of life we were in, notably youth, is a thwarting of the natural movement, so also is using Thanatos to avoid connecting to the new phase a perversion of the life process. Some people on reaching their fifties literally plummet into death and morbidity, and lose all contact with life-giving forces. One fifty-year-old woman declared that she had no fear of death at all; it would be, she said, a relief from the agony of actually getting old. Others in the grip of Thanatos experience feelings of bitterness and betrayal, a sense that life has cheated them, and feel there is no point in doing anything because they are going to die anyway. So cynicism and despair, along with envy of young people, are the signs of somebody falling into the darkness of Thanatos without any sense of its companion instinct of Eros. Just as one can fall in love, one can also fall into destructiveness.

Of course it is difficult to know how to sustain the life force of Eros in the light of the awareness of one's inevitable death. It's a paradox: how does one get connected to ultimately being disconnected? How do we harness Eros into the service of Thanatos and use the energy of connection to help us to begin the task of moving towards our own death without being overwhelmed by despair? Success in this struggle involves a rite of passage which will be the subject of a further chapter. Suffice it to say for the present that it is the capacity to be aware of the interplay of the life and death forces, as Freud said, "that is the meaning of the evolution of civilisation", and indeed, I would add, of the evolution of the individual. In Erik Erikson's terms, the holding of the opposites in consciousness constitutes integrity, which he sees as the final goal of adult development.[3] Undoubtedly the ultimate secret to this integration is the acceptance of our personal death, and in this sense we could consider dying and death as a developmental task in itself. Jung provides a rich and highly relevant comment on this theme of the inevitable movement towards death in an article entitled "The Soul and Death" when he says, "The curve of life is like the parabola of a projectile which, disturbed from its initial state of rest, rises and then returns to a state of repose".[4] A little later on, he says:

> From the middle of life onward, only he remains vitally alive who is ready to *die with life*. For in the secret hour of life's midday the parabola is reversed, death is born. The second half of life does not signify ascent, unfolding, increase, exuberance, but death, since the end is its goal. The negation of life's fulfilment is synonymous with the refusal to accept its ending. Both mean not wanting to live, and not wanting to live is identical with not wanting to die. Waxing and waning make one curve.[5]

Jung's metaphor of a parabola is most apt and brings

into sharp focus our distress at passing the peak of the curve. Yet so often, despite the unavoidable momentum of the descent, we cling with our finger-nails to the peak and continue to look back to it even when we have well and truly begun the descent. The fact is that like a projectile flying towards its goal, life does end in death and the ascent and zenith are only steps in the journey towards the goal. We would be most concerned if a young person refused to accept opportunities for growth and refused to embrace the ascending curve and get on with living. Youth suicide is so profoundly distressing because it violates the natural movement of ascent. Why then should we not be concerned when an individual in the mid-fifties refuses the descent? As Jung again said in the same article, "It is just as neurotic in old age not to focus upon the goal of death as it is in youth to repress fantasies which have to do with the future".[6] But repress we do, both collectively and individually, and our reflex response to the descent is initially one of denial which some people continue, one suspects, to the very end. Such an attitude of denial negates the view that a conscious death is an accomplishment which by the mid- to late fifties certainly ought to be something we are working towards. To see death simplistically as the negation of life is to bring to this transition of dying fearful, neurotic views that are determined by an outer, youthful, materialistic and secular perspective. Hence the vital importance of the shift in the centre of gravity that must be consciously engaged in as part of the fifties transition. To repeat myself, whilst Eros is vital, it is no more vital than Thanatos; the need to live, be connected, must be balanced against the goal of death and the need to be disconnected. To choose to identify exclusively with one or other of these archetypal energies is a form of perversion, change requires a balance of holding on and letting go. What often gets in the way of this integration of Eros and Thanatos is the refusal to embrace and accept the separation from the previous phase. Separation is a form of death and consequently it is often defended against by denial. But such a refusal to hear the call to continue to develop can only lead to the polar opposite of generativity that Erikson speaks of—that is, stagnation and ultimately despair.[7] As the ancient alchemist declared, "Only that which is first separated can be joined together". That is, there can be no integration without separation, since separation forms the first phase of any transition and is the prerequisite for initiation into the next stage of life. It is to the details of this process that we now turn in order to explore the difficulties and gains that are part and parcel of the fifties transition.

---

1   Sigmund Freud (1930), "Civilisation and its Discontents", *Penguin Freud Library* vol. 12, Penguin, Harmondsworth, 1985, p. 314.
2   Sigmund Freud (1915), "On Attitudes toward Death", *Standard Edition* vol. 14, Hogarth Press, London, 1958, pp. 289–300.

3   Erik Erikson, *Childhood and Society*, Norton, New York, 1950, pp. 231–2.
4   C.G. Jung (1934), "The Soul and Death", *Collected Works* vol. 8, Routledge & Kegan Paul, London, 1989, p. 406.
5   ibid.
6   ibid.
7   Erikson, op. cit., p. 232.

3

Rite of Passage

SEPARATION AND MOURNING

The process of changing from one social status to another has been broadly defined as initiation. Culture after culture records the rituals that go with such a change in status, rituals that are often bound up with biological rhythms and in pre-technological societies with meteorological rhythms. The change of status from child to adult in our society is marked when a young person is eighteen and/or twenty-one by such rites of passage as a twenty-first birthday party, the acquiring of a driving licence, entitlement to consume alcohol in public places and the right to vote. Marriage is another rite of passage that we are familiar with, conferring a change of status from single to married. For the gay community, "coming out" has the qualities of a rite of passage accompanying a transition from one socially defined sexual orientation to another. Such rites of passage, often institutionalised in ceremonial form, accompany us throughout our lifetime from birth to the ultimate ritual of a funeral. We need these markers, these rites, to consciously and explicitly make a public declaration and thereby give public weight to the major turning points of our lives.

This public declaration legitimises an individual's change of status, facilitating acceptance of the newly acquired status and the roles that go with it. The same reasoning applies to rituals that are bound up with meteorological rhythms, so harvest festivals denote a change of state from one season to the next. In ancient Ireland, Samhain, the end of summer and the beginning of winter, was a central festival occasion that involved rituals for ensuring the supply of food throughout the long, hard, barren winter.

As we shall see, society does not provide a rite of passage for people entering middle or old age. On the contrary, it systematically ignores this transition, focusing further ahead on the already aged. Again we can see the presence of a collective denial operating here, a denial of the process of ageing and the need to publicly embrace a new status in society, that of being pre-elderly. As I said in the previous chapter, we have vehemently resisted facing our own ageing because we link it to frightening prospects of frailty, dependence, decrepitude and death, all things we would prefer to deny. The net effect of this collective denial is that we have no socially recognised or legitimate role to accompany the change of status that comes with reaching one's fifties. There is a public silence, a gap, in which people can find themselves chronically stuck without any guidelines as to what it means to be a fifty-year-old in our society. Fundamentally it is a liminal state between being young and being old, a state of betwixt and between.

Thus anxieties about being all spent, feelings of invisibility and despair and a pervasive sense of futility can all rush into the vacuum left by the lack of a socially sanctioned change of status and role to accompany being in one's fifties. This leaves a person with the heavy burden of sorting out for themselves how they wish to be, whereas in most other transitions the rite of passage explicitly spells out certain expectations about the type of behaviours that should accompany the change in status. These expectations are a reflection of the underlying archetypal structure of transition, and being part of the collective psyche, they can help to ease an individual's existential angst concerning the change in status. At a time of ambiguity and uncertainty where no clear expectations are defined, people often find that the skills they have so painstakingly acquired are suddenly much less relevant than previously. This can result in a regression to earlier and less helpful behaviours in an attempt to deal with the anxiety.

The fact that we need help by way of a rite of passage with major life transitions is clearly evident in the multitude of initiation ceremonies in so-called primitive societies. Australian Aborigines provide fine examples of initiation rituals denoting a young boy's passage into manhood. These initiation ceremonies involve the symbolic process of death and renewal as well as circumcision and the receiving of sacred knowledge. The ceremonies exclude all women—indeed, the initial step is to take the boy from his mother, whereupon she responds as if he has died; and following his return, some time later, the women shed tears of joy, as if the grave has given up its dead. Such rituals represent an ancient system of spiritual instruction and underline the necessity of separation as a prelude to receiving these instructions, followed by a return with the change of status from boyhood to manhood.

Within the Christian tradition we can see the existence of initiation rites in such ceremonies as baptism and confirmation. These ceremonies often include a change in name and symbolise the process of death and rebirth. Marriage is another typical rite of passage that spells out what is expected with the change of status. These rites of passage protect the emotional well-being of the initiate insofar as they ensure a recognition of psychological development, and the necessity of separation leading to acceptance of the new status and the obligations that it brings.

Perhaps then it is understandable why the transition of the fifties extracts such a heavy psychological burden; in one's soul there exist profound and disturbing rumblings of the change, yet the existence of change is either denied or trivialised. One of Carl Jung's basic dictums was that the failure to fulfil developmental tasks was an important cause of emotional disturbance. He held the view that if the archetypal desire to engage in individuation (or the movement towards wholeness) is thwarted, neurosis is the inevitable result. When change is demanded and yet no helpful initiation rituals or rites of passage exist to provide guidelines, then fear and anxiety must dominate, calling into operation defences that can alter the very personality itself. How often has one heard it said of a man going through the mid-life crisis that "it is as if he is another person". psycho-therapy can, at times like this, play an invaluable role in freeing the natural instinctual desire to continue to develop and embrace the next developmental task, by providing a rite of passage. Indeed, in my experience this is the role psychotherapists are often called upon to perform—that is, to act as secular priests in a rite of passage that has become stuck or even aborted through one means or another. At these times a psychotherapist has to be flexible enough to suspend theoretical assumptions about childhood experiences being the cause of symptoms and be prepared to embrace the ancient Greek role of a *therapeia*, or secular priest or priestess, and help to initiate the client into an age-appropriate status. To adhere rigidly to early childhood perspectives in working with a fifty- to sixty-year-old client is to impose an inappropriate and unhelpful framework on the process. This is not to suggest that earlier patterns are not present, as indeed they clearly are, but rather to emphasise the need to start with the reality in which the client finds him or herself, and to allow for a desire in the human psyche to go forward as well as back. One also needs to allow for the reality of the life transition a person is in, which in the fifties to sixties can include the issue of their own death. Perhaps this is why the psychoanalyst Peter Hildebrand, who spent a considerable number of years working in a psychodynamical way with older clients, expressed the following wish:

> If I had to lay out a therapeutic plan for the future, I would at once ensure that we had a cadre of trained therapists who were capable of developing and deepening our understanding of later life and its problems. What is needed is greater public recognition of the emerging importance of the years between fifty and seventy-five which the French have christened the "Third Age".[1]

The fifties transition is an intricate and complex process of enormous variety to which the appropriate therapeutic response is to try and create the necessary space and climate in which the individual can explore the meaning of the experience. The very absence of some archetypally shaped or informed rite of passage into one's fifties in part accounts for the tremendous variation in the experience. What follows in this book is an attempt, not to provide an explication of a particular rite of passage, nor to deny its complexity and variability. The aim of this book is to share thoughts from people in their fifties in the hope that this will at least provide some markers of the experience that might contribute to a conscious recognition of the process. The appropriate starting point for this is to return to the earlier comments about the ubiquitous nature of loss at this stage of life and to place this loss within the broader context of a transition and rite of passage.

It was Arnold van Gennep in *The Rites of Passage* (1909)[2] who first identified the common structure which underlies all rites of, passage. Since this time his theory has informed numerous cross-cultural studies of the process of initiation. Two contemporary scholars who have developed van Gennep's original proposal are the anthropologist Victor Turner and the mythologist Joseph Campbell. The basic paradigm, which is linked by mythologists such as Campbell to the idea of an heroic undertaking, is a three-stage process of separation, initiation and return. Within the mythological tradition the hero (or heroine) is usually endowed from birth with extraordinary gifts and ability and has to leave his home, or homeland, to fulfil his destiny. Their destiny also demands that he (or she) undergoes a difficult and at times perilous journey, dealing with monsters and other life-threatening events and culminating in the heroic figure overcoming all difficulties and returning to the homeland a transformed person. Myth after myth depicts this journey, with the heroic figure becoming a special figure in the community as a result of the initiation. For women this heroic journey can sometimes be more appropriately depicted by the symbol of a spiral where the journey involves a circular movement that deepens awareness which constitutes the initiation. As part of this initiation and return, the heroic figure sometimes undertakes the significant role of mediator between the world of mortals and the world of gods. He or she has a foot in both camps, so to speak, the mortal world and the divine, the known and the unknown, the material and the immaterial. Within the Greek mythological tradition, the story of Perseus" slaying of the Gorgon who is located at the edge of the world is but one example. Heracles slaying the Hydra and the Nemean lion is another. Within the Irish mythological tradition, the heroic figure is the warrior Cuchulainn; he leaves his home at five years of age to become a famous warrior, slays monsters, journeys to the other world, confronts the dark warrior goddess and returns to Ulster to marry his beloved Emer. These mythological stories narrate the universal heroic process of change, of movement towards a higher and more evolved level of consciousness. In psychological terms the heroic achievement could be seen as the capacity to hold opposites in a conscious relationship with each other. But the first critical step of any heroic journey of enlightenment is an unequivocal separation.

In a somewhat more remote world, that of alchemy, these same three stages of separation, initiation and return form a central theme. The three phases are the *nigredo* or the black of separation; *albedo*, the confrontation and joining of opposites symbolised by white; and the *rubedo*, or red phase, in which the outcome of integration is to produce the philosopher's stone. Alchemy, contrary to biased twentieth-century scientific thinking, was not entirely the domain of charlatans trying to make gold, although no doubt some did exist; rather it was composed of philosopher–scientists who were trying to work out how to perfect themselves through experiments designed to perfect matter and produce gold. They were working in two parallel realities at the same time, believing that if they could work out the process of perfecting matter and making gold, they could then apply these principles to perfecting the human soul. A separating out of the various materials was a vital step in this process. According to some alchemical writers, separation was preceded by a stage called *mortificatio* or death, also sometimes referred to as *putrefactio* or putrefaction, rotting. Paracelsus, a sixteenth-century alchemist, and one of the most famous, said, "Putrefaction is of so great efficacy that it blots out the old nature and transmutes everything into another nature, and bears another fruit. All living things die in it, all dead things decay and then all these dead things regain life".[3]

Putrefaction, which belongs to the *nigredo* phase, is associated with death, decomposition and the breaking down of solid matter. Worms usually accompany the decomposition process, and within the modern psyche worms symbolise putrefaction and death occurring in the unconscious, as the necessary prelude to a renewal or rebirth.

Anne, a woman approaching fifty, dreamt that she was walking with her two sons (in the dream they were eight and twelve years of age). She recalled feeling enormously proud of them in the dream and stopping every now and then to hug and kiss them. The dream continues:

Then I remember leaving the younger one at school and walking down the road where I live. I stopped and watched a large earthworm, which had begun to move when I touched it gently to see if it was alive. It became huge and multiplied into one hundred worms thick and twenty metres long. It was still the one worm. I watched it move towards a tree. It was going faster and faster. As I rushed around the tree the weather, which had been sunny, changed. It darkened and started to rain. A storm was threatening in the background. Then from behind the tree arrived a bridal or wedding party. The bride and groom were from a community in which I grew up. I asked the bride and groom whether they had not already been married and they said no. I was amazed, because they had lived together for fifteen to twenty years and raised a family . . .

Without going into the biographical details of the dreamer, suffice it to say that her early childhood had been rigid and had robbed her of a sense of self-worth.

At the time of the dream she had been divorced for some years and was a single mother. The opening scene depicts attachment, followed by separation and then the appearance of the worm followed by a "change in the weather" and darkness. She was unconsciously sensing the unfolding separation from her children and the reminder that part of her had separated off from conscious development around the age of eight, the age at which she leaves the younger child in the dream. But we see that the separation, followed by the mortification symbol of the worm and then the darkness, brings her to a different place, a place of growth marked by the tree, and the emergence of a union of opposites symbolised by the bridal party. The dream reveals that whilst she has been married externally for fifteen to twenty years, the internal "marriage" of her opposite qualities of the masculine and the feminine was just about to begin. But this perception of change being symbolised by the change in weather only occurs because in the first place she touched and then followed the worm, a symbol of decay, decomposition, fertility and renewal. It is a dream that depicts very clearly the first two parts of any transitional process, the separation and initiation, the *nigredo* and *albedo*, with the *nigredo* symbolising the death of a particular aspect or stage of psychic life. This death often involves the immersion of oneself into the darkness of the unconscious as a prelude to the renewal. It is in the darkness that the seed germinates. As one alchemical text states,

As the grain of wheat sown in the earth putrefies before it springs up into new growth or vegetation, so our Magnesia being sown the Philosophic Earth, dies and corrupts, that it may conceive itself anew.[4]

Thus the first stage of the fifties transition, like every other transition, is a separation which is evoked or called into being by the presence of death or dying in some form. Death, and the awareness of death, is the catalyst for growth and renewal and hearing the call of death, or Thanatos, begins the first stage of the opus. Linda's situation provides a clear example of this process. At the time of our discussion she was in her early fifties, had been married for over thirty years and had three children. Throughout most of her married life she had continued to work. She experienced two significant deaths during the year after she turned fifty. First a very close older friend suicided, which shattered her and left her with a feeling of deep remorse. Six months later her much-loved father died. In the year following this death she was able to describe how she gradually found herself both yearning and able to be alone and reflect, whereas prior to that it had been a life of intense and busy involvement with others. But death called her back into herself, called her to reclaim what she had lost—and now, after over thirty years of marriage, she was planning to separate and pursue in a more complete way her own life, one previously foregone in the service of others.

Paradoxically it is often this very experience of separation that we find unbearable, since it conveys with chilling and compelling clarity that losses have to be incurred and accepted as part of the process of change. Nevertheless there are clearly negative consequences for not embracing and enduring the separation, negative consequences for refusing the heroic call to continue our development. These, as asserted by Jung, are often expressed in neurotic fears and obsessions, and very often in a pathological, narcissistic absorption in one's self. These neurotic patterns bring a certain fixity and rigidity to the person, alienating them from themselves and others and acting as barriers against transition. The problem with separation and the inevitable loss which is entailed is that it opens us up to, or exposes us to, the force of Thanatos, the instinctual drive of disconnection associated with death. This awakening of Thanatos can obliterate, albeit often only temporarily, the life force or Eros. In these moments life is literally not worth living, and finding any sense of connection to anyone or anything can prove to be an almost impossible task. If the black of the *nigredo* and putrefaction sets in . . . then life is felt to be really rotten.

The psychological state that accompanies profound loss is mourning and grief, a process eloquently articulated early in the twentieth century by Sigmund Freud and one that has continued to play a striking role in the theory of psychoanalysis, particularly through the work of such people as John Bowlby. The natural process of mourning is aborted when we cannot accept loss and separation, yet it is this very process that enables renewal to occur. Mourning is the dark ground in which the seed is buried. Yet throughout the discussions I had with people in their fifties, one thing that stood out was the pain of letting go, of separating from aspects of the past, in particular one's youth, and immersing oneself in how really sad it felt. Yet it was equally clear that in those individuals who had experienced death around the late forties or early fifties, whether through a parent or peer death, or maybe a life-threatening illness of their own, or a consciousness of their own death, were more inclined to hear the call and to let go. Confrontation with the death instinct can at the same time mobilise the life instinct.

Jenny was rising fifty-one when I interviewed her. She had been divorced for over twenty years. Her adult children, whom she had raised by herself, had left home and she now lived alone. Jenny was a markedly intro-verted person who had been "properly" brought up; the entire emphasis from her mother was on appearances. The effect of this was to drive any sense of her own self completely underground, and she had developed over the years an over-polite façade which was primarily aimed at seeking approval. She was able to express her terror that if she were really herself, whatever that might have meant, she would risk not only being rejected but being annihilated. Then shortly after turning fifty, her only brother became seriously ill and subsequently died.

The effect of this death was to call herself, her true self, out from behind the mask of appearances—her brother's death literally reignited the spark of self. This took the form of returning to the theatre and taking part in plays, something which she had described as being completely natural. Here death, painful as the loss was, mobilised Eros, and she was able to begin to reconnect to her more authentic self, which when I last saw her was at least competing with the persona and one felt would finally win out in a few years. The awareness of death forces recognition of one's age and mortality, which in turn has the effect of awakening Thanatos from his slumber. Thanatos' twin brother is Somnos the god of sleep, and many people remain asleep or unaware of their own death. But as I have just mentioned, it is the very awakening of consciousness to one's death that provides the call for the heroic journey of the fifties, a journey that involves in the first place separation from our known and fixed views of ourselves. This represents death to the ruling aspects of the psyche, the conscious sense of who we are, (which in alchemy was often depicted as a dying king). The *mortificatio* phase heralds the necessary separation, and this brings with it the loss and the need to grieve for that which is lost.

We tend to think of mourning in the context of bereavement and funerals, so it may seem a little odd to use this word in relation to life transitions. But as Freud pointed out in his pioneering work on mourning and melancholia, "Mourning is regularly the reaction to the loss of a loved person, or to the loss of some abstraction which has taken the place of one, such as one's country, liberty, an ideal and so on".[5]

The "so on" at fifty-plus, as has already been mentioned, involves several things, the primary one being an ideal sense of one's youth and the associated loss of physical prowess and attractiveness. The fifties losses involve the loss of reproductive capacity at menopause for women and the lowering of sexual drive and performance in men at what has been termed the male menarche. There is the loss of opportunity in the workplace and ultimately of work itself, alongside the loss of parental function as children leave home, and not uncommonly the loss of one's parents at the same time. There can be an evocative reminder of the dependency that comes with age in facing the necessary care of one's aged and often frail and senile parents. A further loss, one that usually occurs for the first time now, is the untimely death of one's contemporaries. At or around thirty-five to forty-five some people experience the death of a parent, a loss that can evoke the "mid-life crisis". But at fifty-plus it is the death of one's peers that brings home with unequivocal starkness one's own mortality.

All of these losses must be mourned—a task that includes confronting Thanatos within ourselves. This is so because our notions of death are shaped and coloured by the destructive feelings that form part of Thanatos. Any encounter with death through parents, peers, or the awareness of one's own death re-awakens Thanatos and compels a re-examination of oneself, in particular one's destructiveness towards oneself and others. But for the moment the first task is the acceptance of the separation and losses that are incurred from fifty years on.

The first phase of mourning is characterised by a preoccupation, indeed at times an obsession, with what is lost. The grieving person experiences repeated and painful disappointment and a persistent feeling of anxiety derived from the sense of separation. The thought of what and who we have lost occurs and recurs with painful regularity. This in turn evokes the strongest of urges to recover it, an urge that is most frequently accompanied by violent swings of mood between anger and profound sadness. These efforts to recover continue in spite of the often blatant fruitlessness of the pursuit. Other emotions we experience at this phase in the mourning are feelings of helplessness and hopelessness as the awesome sense of inevitability dawns, despite our often adamant refusal to accept it. The feelings at this stage do not come just from turning fifty, they find their origins in our earliest experiences of loss and are repeated and echoed in the losses one is experiencing at fifty-plus. The anguish we feel in connection with powerful losses is associated with a despairing cry for love to ameliorate the horror of our own demise. The baby's cry, for example, is in one sense a cry of survival and sorrow that biologically is aimed at bringing adults to assist. But what happens to this cry of despair at fifty or so? Who hears it? Who can respond? And have we lost all belief that it would make any difference? We cannot, in our society, openly cry to express the anguish we feel about getting old. Indeed we're not encouraged even to talk about it. No, we have to go on pretending that it is wonderful to be fifty, life is just opening up, etc., etc. Such attitudes reflect a manic defence against the profundity of the sadness. But how many people in their fifties cry in the night as they lie in bed, sleepless, and feel the horror of their own worst and destructive thoughts and the gut-wrenching sadness of their loss? How many people in their fifties have not awoken at night with recurring thoughts of their death, future illness, fear of Alzheimer's disease, the loss of sexual attractiveness, concerns about their ageing menopausal bodies, balding heads, deteriorating skin, etc., etc., and have not as a result felt like crying, with an aching need to recover those things that are lost?

The inability to mourn usually reflects an unwilling-ness to endure this very anguish and to experience the feelings of weakness and vulnerability that come with it. This in part I think is one reason why men find it more difficult to mourn than women—they cannot bear the sense of vulnerability that mourning brings. The pro-found sense of hopelessness, despair and futility are in part the consequence of Thanatos, or the destructive impulse, being directed inward against ourselves as we struggle to stay connected and Thanatos struggles to disconnect us.

WOMEN AND THE LOSS OF YOUTH

Amongst the people I interviewed, it was very clear that for women body changes, often crystallised in menopause, were the first unequivocal signs of the loss of youth. Sometimes cessation of menstruation was less significant than subtle changes in the body, in particular the skin: woman after woman spoke with sadness of perceived change in the tone, texture and colour of her skin as if it was in some way the boundary between youthfulness and age. The body is the vehicle for conveying the first undeniable awareness of no longer being youthful. Little wonder, then, that it is also the increasing object of cosmetic surgery. Along with changes in the living boundary of the skin are other observations of greying hair, for example, and changes in body shape bringing an unwelcome realisation of the necessity to change one's clothing style. For many women the decision to let the grey hair show is a ritualistic moment of letting age through. So the attractive, sexually enticing clothes that reveal bodies and the female form as part of courtship rituals have now to be nostalgically glimpsed and passed by, just as is the experience of youth.

What struck me with a forceful clarity was the profound difference between men and women in acceptance of the inevitability of body changes. By and large men go into full-blown denial, continuing to delude themselves that they are permanently somewhere between thirty-five and forty-five and still irresistibly attractive to women. It leaves open the thought that despite the obvious complexity of menopause, whether natural or induced, it is a profound marker of the transition, a marker that men do not have. For a woman it heralds the end of reproduction and the end of one way of being a woman, the death of one's maidenhood and motherhood and the initiation into the role of wise old woman, or crone.

Clearly women's responses to menopause will be highly variable. There is pressure to consider the process in a stereotyped manner, especially with the growing medicalisation of menopause and the push for hormone replacement therapy. Germaine Greer in her book *The Change* asserts that the menopausal woman is the prisoner of a stereotype and will not be rescued from it until she has begun to tell her own story. A little later she states, "If fifty year old women were visible in our culture we would know that every climacteric is different; it is only our ignorance that implies that all menopausal women are enduring the same trials and responding in the same way".[6]

The very word "climacteric", a more correct term than "menopause", is interesting in itself since it is derived from the Greek word *klimakter*, which means important step or stage, critical period. Yet it is a critical transition, or step, that has remained relatively undiscussed, even tabooed. There is no recognised rite of passage, it is an intensely private experience, yet an undeniably significant one. Germaine Greer is perhaps a little extreme, but nevertheless captures the experience of many women when she says, "The shame that she felt at the beginning of her periods is as nothing compared to the long drawn out embarrassment occasioned by their gradual stopping".[7]

It is difficult to ascertain with any clarity the many factors that must contribute to this sense of shame. But what one can say is that shame, unlike guilt, is socially induced, created from outside. In other words one is *made* to feel ashamed. Amongst the women I spoke with, a possible source of shame was firstly the fact that unlike so many of a woman's other transitions, such as birth, marriage and childbearing, all of which are regarded as fulfilling important social functions and hence have rituals attached to them to publicly acknowledge their value to society, menopause involves no one other than the woman herself, and this contributes a certain element of invisibility and secrecy. This is on top of the growing sense one has of becoming less visible with age anyway. This feeling of invisibility as part of their ageing experience was something many women raised in discussions with me.

Women who had measured their validity according to the amount of male attention they received found menopause most painful, catapulting them into invisibility. These women, who had throughout their lives relied on their sexual attractiveness and beauty to define who they were, experienced menopause not as a change, or even "the change", but as a death sentence. It is particularly painful for women coming into their fifties who find themselves without a partner, if having a partner has been an important desire for them. Menopause and the heralding of being in the third stage of womanhood, the crone stage, signified and confirmed for them their worst fears of ending up alone. As well as bringing an awful confirmation of their great fear of being alone, ageing underlined and consolidated the many disappointments they had experienced in past relationships with men. These disappointments had often been made bearable in the past by the hope that there would still be future opportunities of meeting men. These feelings are succinctly captured by Simone de Beauvoir in *The Second Sex*:

> Long before the eventual mutilation, woman is haunted by the horror of growing old . . . she has gambled much more heavily than the man on the sexual values she possesses; to hold her husband and assure herself of his protection, it is necessary for her to be attractive, to please . . . What is to become of her when she no longer has any hold on him? This is what she anxiously asks herself, as she helplessly looks on at the degeneration of this fleshly object that she identifies with herself.[8]

De Beauvoir wrote these words at forty-one, long before her physical attractiveness had declined, so they cannot accurately reflect the reality of her own situation.

Rather it is her last line that reveals the source of her distress and dejection and that is where she explicitly states her identity as a woman being tied to what she terms the "fleshly object". In acceding to this, a woman is allowing herself to be defined by the patriarchal world that will leave her feeling worthless and invisible at and after menopause.

But this view is not shared by many other women whose sense of being and identity has been derived from several sources both inner and outer. For these women the goddess is a triple one—maiden, mother and crone—and not a single goddess of sexuality and physical attractiveness. Women who have derived their sense of themselves from a wider base than just the outer world also tend to be individuals who have processed other major changes in their lives. This will include the critical one from maidenhood to motherhood and the changing relationships with their own children. These fundamental changes, all involving loss and separation at some point, prepare many women for the menopausal change and they are therefore receptive to the understanding that loss and change is the essential quality of human experience. For women who have not had children, no matter how consciously they regard themselves as having made the choice not to, menopause removes the choice completely and the possibility of the experience of giving birth is foregone with a powerful sense of finality, indeed a death-like finality.

Yet this very process of the climacteric involving the

death of one aspect of feminine being, reproduction, is at the same time a process of birth itself. It can be the birth of her crone self, or the rebirth of her maiden self in an older matured form. Loss of fertility is a loss at one level only, the physical; it does not mean a loss of desire and fulfilment. But it clearly demands a willingness to mourn for the loss of oneself as a young reproductive woman if one is to reach the third stage of self, that knows and accepts the eternal cycle of birth, life and death—a self that can make the passage from outer to inner, from body into soul, from persona towards self. Presumably this is what Germaine Greer means in the quotation given earlier when she says that a menopausal woman remains prisoner of a stereotype until such time as she can tell her own story, speaking from the true self rather than a socially constructed one—a construction that has by and large been determined by the demands of others, predominantly children and husbands. Yet optimism and embracing of a reborn self is vulnerable to sabotage and abortion from within the woman herself, and also from the external patriarchal world in which she resides. The difficulty that women experience in sustaining their own rebirth is most clearly seen in dreams in which the symbol of a new baby often depicts the reborn self that we have been discussing. Joan was just approaching fifty when she had the following dream:

I find my baby but I can't remember where. She is tiny but beautiful and very alive and smiling and bright-eyed.

I hold her with one hand against my chest. I can't remember what happens next but I've gone away to do something and I come over some grass on a lawn and find a little baby wrapped in swaddling clothes lying on the grass. She is still smiling. Later again I come back to her and find that she has been dying. She is the size of my hand and dehydrated. I wonder if it is too late. I put my finger under a garden tap and she sucks my finger and I think she is alive. I give her more from my finger and she starts to revive. I see a baby's bottle in front of me full of water. This will sustain her I think . . .

There is much one could say about this dream but what it clearly depicts is the difficulty this woman, and many women, find in knowing how to sustain their new growth. In part this difficulty reflects the simple fact of lack of practice, particularly where the demands of being a mother and wife have dulled a woman's sensibilities to her own needs, her inner self. In this dream we see the dreamer doesn't really know even where the new sense of self has come from and after welcoming it, she goes off to do something else. The beginning of menopause, ironically, can be the moment of conception of this new sense of self, but a woman can be unaware of the link and respond to it by racing off and doing more tasks, in a sort of flight into pragmatism. The result is that the reborn sense of self literally dehydrates, runs out of feeling and is threatened with extinction. Fortunately this dreamer, at least unconsciously, revived the newborn part of herself with water, a symbol for feeling, and indeed towards the end of the dream she has consolidated her care by now coming across a bottle full of water.

Whilst there is this inner threat of abortion of the newborn self, there also exists an outer threat. The patriarchal outer world holds fears about crones: they are seen as the keepers of secrets about birth and death, and as having the strength to speak of both these things. This is a confronting reminder to the triumphant masculine world of the inevitability of loss, a loss that the masculine world usually does not wish to know about. Germaine Greer calls this fear of the crone "anophobia", meaning an irrational fear of old women. This third stage of womanhood, the crone phase, threatens men also with the possibility of not being able to control women, hence the need to dismiss and denigrate, as when someone is said to behave "like an old woman" or to be "an old bag". The contempt in such phrases is, I suggest, forged out of fear. But without a rite of passage to validate them at such transitional times as menopause, women are vulnerable. They are likely to internalise this derision and believe it to be true of themselves. Self-recrimination can take hold of a woman and in the grips of Thanatos she can "forget" that she is entering a new and profoundly important stage of her life where freedom from this derision can also be found. It is a stage where the call to move from a false, outer-directed to a true, inner-directed self can often be heard clearly for the first time. This is a theme that we shall take up in more detail in connection with the "empty nest" phase of a woman's life.

MEN AND THE LOSS OF YOUTH

If the woman who reaches menopause is under threat of derision by the patriarchal world and its values, then one can readily appreciate how complex the loss of youth must be for males, who are both the inventors and upholders of patriarchal values. The effect for men is that their sense of identity is formed and bound by prevailing social expectations. The average man's sense of identity revolves around status, power, success, action, knowledge, physical strength and sexual prowess. Even a cursory list of these qualities immediately alerts one to their essentially outer-directed nature. The end result is that most men are more stereotyped, more predictable and less individuated than women. The prize for men is not individuality but power and status—i.e. affirmation from the outer world that not only are they somebody, a proper man, but that they actually exist. Of course there are many men who do not share these values. Very often these are creative men who exist on the margin of society as mavericks, foregoing the satisfaction of social approval. However, such men are clearly the exception, not the rule, and the majority of men unconsciously and without any reflection continue to assess themselves by the traditional outer values of sex, power and status.

If the menopausal woman who has restricted her sense of identity to the physical realm of attractiveness to men finds menopause a serious threat to her sense of well-being, then how much more powerful must be the threat to males who have by and large exclusively defined themselves by outer factors? The loss of youth in men seems also to threaten the loss of identity per se. Little wonder, then, that men resist the ageing process with more vigour than women. At some level of the psyche, age threatens a nothingness, perhaps a no-*thing-ness*, annihilation, a void—a threat that is enough to drive a man back out into the world of action with renewed gusto.

It is at mid-life that most men get their first glimpse of age, a glimpse that is given usually through the dual lens of body changes and the bursting into youthful adulthood of adolescent children. An adolescent, particularly a teenage son, serves to remind the average mid-life man of the brutal fact that he is on the other side of youth, energy and vitality. But after a temporary period of disillusion and depression the mid-life male simply picks up his cudgels and determinedly sets out to re-conquer the world, even if he has redefined what constitutes the world. The hero of mid-life usually re-commits himself to triumphing over uncertainty, dependency and vulnerability and sees the source of his ills as lying outside himself in either family, marriage or work. At thirty-five to forty he still has a sufficiently youthful body and mind, plus the perception of sufficient or indeed ample time, to re-ignite lost youth and compete more than adequately with the younger brigade snapping at his heels. In the realm of sex he still sees himself as attractive and sexually strong, and in his erotic fantasy life he conquers woman after woman.

By fifty, however, the physical realities are at odds with a man's fantasy. The male body loses strength, gets heavier, changes shape; the hair gets thin, skin deteriorates, jowls develop around the jaw and neck; sexual desire wanes, erections are weaker and physical complaints start to increase. The mirror is often actively avoided, unless it is used to create a self-delusion of how youthful and virile one actually looks. On top of all this, work has frequently become repetitious and boring, and a man's career has often begun to peter out regardless of what field he works in. In a sense these are the same issues as arise in mid-life, but in the fifties they are magnified and less amenable to being triumphed over. Since a man does not have the obvious and powerfully symbolic internal benchmark that the cessation of menstruation provides, his losses do not connect him to the inevitable cyclical nature of life. No, for a man, it is loss, loss, and more loss, with little or no sense of an inner fertile space or source to fall back on. It is not that men do not have an inner world, it is rather that in being so outer-directed men have a very limited notion of how to get connected to it. They have had very little, if any, practice, other than the experience of mid-life, and have often come to distrust inner experience.

This is why mid-life stands out as a very important transition, since it gives a man his first adult opportunity to reflect and re-negotiate the identity that was originally firmly set in adolescence and often included his choice of career. How he manages mid-life, as has been mentioned, will provide a reasonably reliable guide as to how he will manage the fifties transition. If he simply had one look and then regressed to action by running back out into the world, the chances are he will try a variation of the same strategy during the fifties. If, on the other hand, he struggled with the meaning of what was happening to him, with the depression and futility he felt, used it as a time of reflection and made some changes in his way of being, the outcome will be different: he is more likely to value feeling and the inner life. A third possibility is that he ignored entirely the disturbance of mid-life, often because he was too busy; one finds that these men usually experience a delayed mid-life crisis at or around fifty years of age.

What lies behind these patterns, for men as for women, is a profound sadness at the loss of one's youth. As we have seen, the appropriate and mature response to this perceived loss is to mourn, to struggle to accept the pain of the loss and the inevitability of change. But this task seems to be more difficult for men than women, perhaps because they find it harder to tolerate being in a position of "weakness" and vulnerability such as mourning entails. As a consequence, the separation from youth is more often than not aborted, with no rebirth emerging.

Denial of ageing constitutes a refusal to hear the call for the heroic adventure of facing and accepting the inevitability of loss and ultimately of one's death. Thus, in Jung's terms, individuation or maturation is thwarted. From a Jungian viewpoint men who deny they are ageing remain puers, or eternal youths, still seeking escape from a reality that they do not wish to acknowledge because it doesn't fit with their fantasies.

Paul is an example of such a man: his life literally came apart between the ages of fifty and fifty-three when his business crashed, resulting in substantial financial loss, and his third marriage broke up. Paul's father had died when he was fifty-one, yet Paul himself when he reached fifty-one had completely denied this fact and remained unconscious of the link between his age and his father's age at death. A consistent fact of life is that as adults we are very influenced, either wittingly or unwittingly, by the age at which our parents died, particularly the same-sex parent. No matter how much one might like to construct rationales for why we will not die at the same age—because we have a different history, different lifestyle, etc., etc.—the psychic reality is that we do expect to die at the same age or earlier. Therefore approaching or reaching the age at which a significant parent died sets up a disturbance in the psyche and acts as a call, indeed a shout, to confront the question of one's own mortality. It is in many senses the initiatory call into the next step of development. But Paul had remained unaware of this call and instead, as was his pattern chose the puer hope of a solution to his unease outside himself in repeated marriages. His energy was spent in seeking ways of achieving immortality rather than facing mortality; in denying age, he was attempting to defy death.

A hallmark of men like Paul is that they persist in and often actively pursue the belief, via gurus and innumerable workshops, that there really is an answer to life. This is a pursuit that keeps them looking anywhere other than within, in some idealised younger female partner, or quasi-magical New Age philosophy or solution. Refusal to hear the call to mourn lost youth frequently results in the outer life falling into tatters as destructive urges are directed towards the self, undermining the healthy regard and love one might have for oneself. The long-term effect of this is that old age will bring despair and self-disgust, not integrity.

Other men refuse to separate from idealised notions of themselves as permanently youthful by behaving as if they are still young. Thus at the earliest signs of ageing they re-immerse themselves in the pursuit of power. We are also witnessing an increase in men seeking cosmetic surgery and hair transplants to maintain the illusion of perpetual youth, since the loss of hair is usually equated with the loss of potency and youth. Concern about potency gets to the core of a male's identity since the penis symbolises power. Hence another solution to the anxiety of ageing is to find a new, preferably younger, lover to confirm one's youth and attractiveness. Here, as in the amazing proliferation of potency clinics, the fervent welcome for Viagra, and the introduction of hormonal treatment for low testosterone levels, we see that men are dealing with the pain of losing youth by external means, not by internal reflection upon their feelings about getting old and ultimately dying. To lose one's sexual potency is for many men in fact a death, the death of a key aspect of a man's identity. (It raises an interesting question, by the way, as to how these men view the women in their lives; I suspect they see women principally as objects of desire.) It's a repetition of the well-worn male pattern of when in doubt take action, resort to technology and machines—a philosophy that keeps men permanently imprisoned in the outer world, completely unprepared for the significant transition into old age and ultimately death.

To return to an earlier theme of Eros and Thanatos, what one can observe in the male preoccupation with sex and sexual potency in connection with getting older is the blocking of Thanatos. The sexualisation of the anxiety aroused by loss of youth signifies the appropriation of Eros into warding off Thanatos. Disconnection from youth is blocked by the eroticisation of loss. Blocked in this way, Thanatos (or the destructive face of it) often finds its way out through other avenues. So the man obsessed with maintaining his power and potency will be vulnerable to obsessive envy of younger people and colleagues in the workplace, which most likely will take the form of denigrating and demeaning them or spitefully blocking opportunities for them to develop.

Another way in which the destructive aspect of Thanatos can emerge when not utilised in the task of disconnection is in the destruction of a marriage, by attacking and demeaning one's often long-standing partner, or simply by withdrawing and being emotionally unavailable. The pursuit of sexual affairs at this time embodies both the destructive face of Thanatos, insofar as they are often exploitative and inappropriate relationships, and yet at the same time they meet the neurotic need to reassure oneself of one's potency. Divorcing one's long-standing marital partner and re-partnering with a younger woman is only minimally about sex and maximally about power, since it often represents a desire to have a dependent, compliant female partner who will not threaten the man's need for dominance and power. Many men fear a loss of control, because it means they will not be able to structure situations in order to avoid contact with their feelings, their sadness, their vulnerability, their neediness—all matters which would shift their centre of gravity from the narcissistic outer self to a connection with the inner, more feminine and compassionate self that Jung has termed the anima.

Finally there is another pattern in men, one which applies equally often to women, and that is to literally fall into the arms of Thanatos and engage in thoroughly self-destructive behaviour. Loss arouses envy, self-hatred, self-persecution and depression—some people obliterate Eros and any love feelings for themselves or others. In certain circumstances the loss of youth evokes rage, or outrage, at one's failings and lost opportunities. This in turn can lead to strong envy of others who appear more powerful, more successful and better off. The hate that is directed inward in these circumstances can be debilitating, and severe depression is a very real possibility, as is self-destructive acting out which can include suicide, alcoholism and the abuse of the body culminating in chronic physical illness. The balance between Eros and Thanatos is both a delicate and critical one, and if one aspect is in the ascendant at the expense of the other, then symptomatic behaviour is the result. Both instincts are needed to enable disconnection from one stage of life and reconnection to the next.

FIFTY OR FIFTEEN?

The loss of youth for both genders evokes changes in identity, since so much of our ego identity is tied up with body. It was Freud who said, "The ego is first and foremost a bodily ego".[9] To slightly rephrase this, one might say that the ego is body long before it is anything else and our sense of "I" is firstly a body sense of "I". Thus disturbances to the body by natural biological processes, injuries, surgery or ageing have a profound effect on how we see ourselves and who we see ourselves as. At fifty-plus there is an obvious and striking parallel to adolescence, not only around the question of "Who am I?" but also in connection with bodily changes. Changes to the body at puberty compel a change of identity from child to young adult, bringing confusion, uncertainty and chaos. At fifty-plus, changes in the body dictate that the same confusion and uncertainty prevail. In one situation it is developing or evolving and in the other it is deteriorating or involuting. The body itself is intrinsically involved in both.

If we accept the parallel between adolescence and the fifties transition, we will not be surprised if some unresolved issues of adolescence re-emerge in the fifties. At any one point in time we may be functioning in a number of different time scales, and biological age is only one of those. There is enough similarity between the experience of being fifty and being an adolescent to evoke the co-existence of the adolescent time scale. Both stages of the life cycle require adjustment to sexual and biological changes and usually shifts in role, including those arising from career changes. Both groups struggle with the question of dependence and independence. For adolescents, and adults in their fifties, there are concerns about financial resources, adolescents worrying about how to get it and later fifties adults worrying about how to keep it. During both periods there is the complex pattern of moving from a two-generational home to a one-generational household. Adolescents have the developmental task of preparing for and ultimately leaving home, late fifties adults have the task of accepting their children's departure and themselves reverting to being a pair. Under these social and biological pressures, old defences and old ways of coping tend to break down, which can precipitate a very real crisis of identity forcing fundamental changes to the way a person sees himself or herself. One way of dealing with the need to separate and simultaneously cope with feelings of attachment along with making the necessary adjustments to sexual and biological changes is to revert to adolescent ways—i.e. to act out rather than contain and reflect upon the struggle. This tendency to act out often finds its origins in unresolved issues from adolescence, especially the early death of a parent and the incessant and usually unmet need for parental approval and emotional availability during adolescence. The awakening of one's own mortality and loss of youth in the fifties literally resurrects earlier losses and deaths. So if a person has experienced the death of a parent around the time of their own puberty then there will be a tendency to deal with this in an adolescent rather than adult manner. This is not to suggest that people are necessarily immature per se, but rather to indicate that we carry within us early wounds to the self from a long time back and when re-awakened we tend to experience all the feelings of that period, including the ways we dealt with them then. At fifty or thereabouts there is a second chance to reflect back on the losses and wounds, to mourn for them, and gradually move from depression and anger to acknowledging the sadness, accepting ourselves and the losses and finally reaching some point of reparation and forgiveness of those who we felt caused our suffering. But this is the orderly process of mourning, a process that we have already seen is often aborted by one's inability or refusal to bear the loss. Some defend against the loss by acting out in sexual and/or aggressive ways, others, as we have already seen, through self-denigrating fantasies of worthlessness culminating in despair.

John was fifty-one at the time of the interview. He had been a very successful businessman and was now divorced with three children, two in their twenties and one a late teenager. His initiation into ageing was via ill-health, a physical complaint that had persisted for many months and was resistant to cure. In this time he had sold his business and was able to express that what was changing for him was his relationship to work and a lessening of his need for power and status. He said quite openly and honestly, that ever since he was a teenager he had fantasised about making a discovery of some sort or having an idea that would make him famous. This yearning, which had clearly not been satisfied by his material success, had driven him through much of his adult life and was once again very strong in him, particularly since he had terminated his business. It was a deep yearning to be recognised as somebody of substance. He had several dreams about not being able to enter water—the ocean, a flooded basement, a river. A problematic relationship with the internal feminine image was another recurrent theme. Both these symbols we might take to represent feelings. The critical point of his history was that his father had died unexpectedly, as John was coming into puberty. He had just passed the exact age at which his father had died and the preceding year had been disturbing, culminating in his desire for a career change. Whilst he willingly reflected on his awareness of ageing, the possibility of death was absent from our discussion. The desire to be famous most likely stemmed from the loss of his father just as he was coming into manhood. Literally it left him without a role model and a source of validation as a man or somebody of worth. His yearning was reawakened around the time he reached the fifty mark and was impairing his capacity to value himself. This will probably only be achieved when he does enter the water, listens to his feelings, and allows himself to know how vulnerable and really sad he feels about the loss of his father. In the meantime, driven by his adolescent issues he seeks to find fame and fortune in the world by acquiring new knowledge and triumphing over uncertainty rather than embracing it. The desire to triumph over uncertainty has a lot to do with the need to control one's life in the hope that we will not be hurt again, rather than it being a simple notion of control per se. But the refusal to embrace uncertainty and let go of control works against mourning, and thereby impairs or inhibits transition into the next stage of adult development.

Another person, Elizabeth, had experienced the

death of her mother through cancer when she was twelve years of age. As a consequence, she had become the mother to her youngest siblings prior to leaving home around eighteen or nineteen. The shadow of her mother's death dominated her psychic life and she found renewal and Eros difficult to sustain. At fifty-eight, she still saw death as a thief and feared her own ageing and death. Self-denigration, an adolescent turning in of self-hatred, pervaded her thoughts and led her into feelings of despair. She yearned to change, but getting connected to an inner image of renewal was very difficult because Thanatos, or disconnection, had a profound grip on her. There probably is no more powerfully determining psychic event than the early loss of a mother; it continues to determine much of one's adult life. The damage can be partly ameliorated when one becomes a parent, but it returns with a vengeance when one reaches the age at which the parent died. The psychic ghost literally comes back to haunt. Many changes had occurred in Elizabeth's life when she reached the age at which her mother died, and she had a pervasive sense of confusion, loss and vulnerability around identity, probably echoing her feelings in adolescence and her response to the death of her mother.

Seeing death as a thief who robs one of life is not uncommon, and it is connected to the experience of feeling that one has not had life. In the terms we have been using so far, it comes from having experienced

Thanatos as the predominant force throughout life rather than Eros. The origins of this imbalance are manifold, beginning with an adverse innate balance between the destructive and constructive drives. Sometimes it comes from an over-strict internal conscience due to religious upbringing or very authoritarian parents. It may also find its origins in an emotionally vulnerable and unavailable mother, or a violent, alcoholic, abusive father. The net result is that the person experiences hatred, anger, despair and pessimism far more than the opposites of love, optimism and hope. Adolescence is a vulnerable time when these tendencies can "set" in the human psyche and substantially affect later adult life. So the experience of an alcoholic father can leave a woman with strong doubts about her self-worth, and reaching fifty can awaken this pain from adolescence, a pain that (as we will discuss shortly) is often stirred by one's own adolescent children leaving home, especially when this coincides with menopause and turning fifty. In families where there has been violence and alcoholism, it is not uncommon to find adolescents leaving home acrimoniously and early. The accumulated heavy loss evokes strong self-recrimination and despair, together with a distinct feeling that death is in fact a thief. The truth is that Thanatos has been robbing them of life throughout their lives. The prospect of their own physical death merely serves to highlight this fact, painfully.

One woman with such a history said she had been an

alcoholic but stopped drinking at fifty as she approached the age at which her father had died from alcoholism. Somehow she had kept enough Eros and self-love intact to turn the tide and end the self-destructive imitation of her father's pattern. Sometimes Eros is kept alive in these situations through sexual affairs through the thirties and forties, but sexualising the loss brings only temporary triumph over it and does not allow it to be worked through. By fifty this is a less-than-productive way of dealing with loss.

Jane was fifty-two at the time of the study and whilst she did not speak of death robbing her, or mention it as a fear, she repeatedly talked of "time running out". She had just reached the age at which her over-idealised father had died, and she had entered menopause. These losses she had dealt with by becoming promiscuous and having several affairs, all of which she had kept secret from her husband. The pattern met important needs: she continued to gain the admiration of the dead idealised father, (one of her lovers had been considerably older than her) and counteracted the feelings of loss of sexual attractiveness that had been awakened by the coming menopause. She described herself as preoccupied with control, which did not seem incorrect, but what she was in fantasy trying to control was death and her own destructiveness, by eroticising it. Here again we have an example of Eros being inappropriately engaged to prevent change, not to connect to it. Much of Jane's behaviour and the way in which she dealt with change echoes the acting-out and the pursuit of admiration from the outside world, characteristic of adolescence. Her strong feeling of "time running out" further indicates an immature level of thinking; there's a fantasy of omnipotence embedded in the idea that one can actually control time, rather than the more adult response of learning to yield to it and embracing the next stage.

Before we leave this important theme of loss of youth we need to return to two earlier points which help us appreciate how powerful early losses can be and how significant they are in our adult lives. First, I said that the way each individual deals with the challenges and anxieties of any one stage will influence his or her capacity to cope with the crises associated with the following stage. This cumulative loss or gain model was first clearly articulated by Erik Erikson in his work *Childhood and Society*. Second, I made the point that it is sheer folly to think we are just one age—in fact we are in several time zones, or ages, at any one point in time. Thus the adult who experiences the early death of a parent carries around inside the sad, bereft young child which makes its presence felt at other times of loss. The validity of these assertions is clearly seen in the case of James, who consulted me for psychotherapy. At the time of the initial contact he was fifty-eight years old, and his presenting problem was that he felt nauseous when physically close to a woman. He elaborated by saying that it only occurred four to six months after the initial period of sexual intimacy. He had divorced his first wife after some twenty years of marriage, and following several short-term relationships he had remarried and had been in that marriage for the past three to four years. The problem of his nausea had pervaded the second marriage and was causing tension, finally resulting in a trial separation. He was able to report that he did not experience this nausea in transitory or casual sexual relationships, it only occurred when the relationship got to the four- to six-month point.

Two things stood out about James: one was his near-obsession with being youthful, his pride in feeling physically fit and young; the second was the extreme difficulty he found in bringing feelings and fantasies or dreams to the sessions. He had undertaken a considerable amount of therapy prior to seeing me, but making any meaningful feeling contact with him, despite the very thoughtful and at times insightful comments that he made, was very difficult.

James revealed that his father had died of an illness when James was five to six years of age. His primary memory was of a sick and debilitated father plus some very early memories of himself as a carefree child playing in the garden alongside his father's business prior to the illness. After his father died he was brought up by his mother under difficult financial circumstances, and his memories were sparse but characterised by a profound sense of deprivation. When he was approaching puberty, his mother developed a debilitating

disease that rendered her virtually immobile and bed-
ridden. He described how from twelve on he and his
sister brought themselves up. He was able to express
some anger around the fact that his father's brothers and
extended family had ignored them following his father's
death. He clearly saw them as potential resources that
could have eased his pain, but for reasons he did not
understand they chose not to be involved.

By any standards this is a very sad history, even
though I cannot convey the depth of sadness and
emotional deprivation James felt in the short account I
have given. He demonstrated, throughout my contact
with him, enormous resistance to exploring his father's
death and his considerable anger and sadness around
this. Instead he displaced all his sadness, seeing his
mother's illness as the cause of his unhappiness and difficulties in relationships. It was not unrelated, of course,
but it is a little too neat to simply see the nausea he felt
towards women being as a result of having a mother
whose body was misshapen and damaged by illness.
However, he had seen several therapists, all of whom,
either wittingly or unwittingly, had provided him with
consolation of this particular story. I felt what he had
was a therapy story and not a history, or his-story, that
found its impetus in the father's death. How could a
little five-year-old boy face the bewilderment and
sadness of a father dying, along with a mother who no
doubt was distraught with her own grief? It seemed to
me that it was symbolically significant that after five

67

to six months the nausea started, thereby parallelling his own unresolved grief at five to six years of age. It was as if something had made him sick and needed to be vomited up. After a period of five to six months in a relationship, attachment begins to develop, and for him this probably brought back the terror of abandonment he must have felt when his father died. However, his focus on his mother's illness prevented any meaningful access to the father's death. The physical image of a crippled mother held in a symbolic sense his own crippled self, one that he had shunned and avoided. His near-obsession with being youthful, extending to his dress, represented a denial of ageing and death. To accept his own age and mortality would have awoken the pain of the five-year-old boy.

James finally chose to discontinue therapy without the issue of his father's death ever being adequately worked through. It was as if he had to leave the "father" (me) this time rather than be left, perhaps on the basis that attack is the best form of defence. The most compelling metaphor capturing the extent to which James was in the grips of his unacknowledged and incomplete mourning was an old house that he had purchased to live in and renovate. He found that he was paralysed by the task and quite unable to get on with the renovation. Renovation and renewal are interchangeable, and the creativity associated with them is only possible when first we acknowledge the death and the loss that goes with it, accept the sadness, and then set about the business of restoring life as a result of the mourning process. Getting old, being in one's fifties, is a little like James' house: our sense of who we are, where we live, is deteriorating, in need of renovation, but first we must assess and accept the extent of the deterioration, the appropriateness of where the renovation should be carried out and then begin the task with a conscious appraisal and not an idealised notion that it will all just happen.

This case, apart from demonstrating how early death of a parent can impede later transitions, raises another point which we will explore in detail further on but which needs comment here—James' marked inability to fantasise or imagine. Since Freud's time it has been well established that incomplete mourning inhibits the development of symbolic or imaginative thought and drives people out into a fixed, concrete literality, away from their imaginative life. Internalising, or developing an internal sense and image of the person who has died or of that which has been lost, is a critical part of the grieving process. Failure to internalise can inhibit the development of our capacity to engage in symbolic thought. This is the very capacity that we need if we are to work through our losses, including the loss of youth, since by being able to think symbolically we can reflect upon the issues, contain them within ourselves and not act them out, or see the cause of our ills as lying outside ourselves. As Hannah Segal states, "Symbol formation is the outcome of loss, it is a creative work involving the pain and the whole work of mourning".[10]

This process of giving the outer event a psychic reality is central to the development of creative life and imaginative thinking, as opposed to the concrete, literal thinking that characterises James' behaviour, which in the long run seeks an outer solution to an inner conflict.

The loss of youth is but one of the powerful outer events that occur when we reach our fifties. Each provides a stimulus or a task, which is always to transform the outer event into psychic material through the process of symbol formation, which in turn provides the opportunity to reflect not project. The next chapter focuses on one of these major outer events, children leaving home.

---

1   P. Hildebrand, *Beyond Mid-Life Crisis*, op.cit., p. 26.

2   A. van Gennep, *The Rites of Passage*, translated by M.B. Vizendom & G.L. Caffee, University of Chicago Press, 1960.

3   *The Hermetic and Alchemical Writings of Paracelsus*, 1:153, edited and translated by A.E .Waite, New York University Books, New York, 1967.

4   M.A. Atwood, *Hermetic Philosophy and Alchemy* (1850), reprint, Julian Press, New York, 1960, p. 115n.

5   S. Freud (1917), "Mourning and Melancholia", *Standard Edition* vol. 14, Hogarth Press, London, 1917, pp. 251–2.

6   G. Greer, *The Change: Women, Ageing and the Menopause*, Hamish Hamilton, London, 1991, pp. 18, 21.

7   ibid., p. 35.

8   S. de Beauvoir, *The Second Sex*, edited and translated by H.M. Parshley, Penguin, Harmondsworth, 1984, pp. 587–8.

9   S. Freud (1923), *The Ego and the Id, Standard Edition* vol. 19, Hogarth
    Press, London, 1962, p. 26.
10 H. Segal, "A Psychoanalytic Contribution to Aesthetics", *International
    Journal of Psychoanalysis* 33, 1952.

4

Marriage, the Empty Nest and the True Self

While the loss of youth evidenced in bodily changes is the most obvious evidence of ageing, and the one we first experience, other arenas of life are also involved in the process of ageing. Whilst body is, as Freud reminded us, intrinsically related to our sense of identity it is not the only source of it, particularly in adult life. Two others that play a substantial part in shaping many people's sense of identity are marriage and work. Moving into the fifties impacts substantially on these realms as we confront a changing sense of self, and this demands the same separating process as the ageing body does from youthful perceptions of ourselves.

One major aspect of the fifties for many individuals is the end of their parenting role when the last child leaves home—the "empty nest" phase—which I will discuss in some detail. There are aspects of this stage in life that are shared by people who have neither been married nor become parents and also those who are not in a long-term relationship: the struggle to stay connected to an inner sense of self, menopause, the emergence of androgyny and an increase in dependency. Several of these are the direct consequence of a reduction in responsibility, either chosen or forced, through such circumstances as early retirement or redundancy. This creates a vacuum and sense of loss of which the empty nest is but one specific, albeit common, version. Because it is such a prevalent experience for individuals in their fifties I have chosen to focus on the empty nest, not only in its own right but also as a vehicle for exploring issues that are more generally applicable regardless of one's marital status.

The empty-nest stage of family life has often been trivialised and dismissed in comments about people now being free to enjoy life. These comments are the manic and denying face of the sad or depressed feelings that often accompany this stage of parenthood. The empty-nest phase is a complex one that involves some very fundamental issues of identity, particularly for women. Fantasies of a renewed youth and freedom, of time to spend, travel, shift house or live in some trendy *caffé latte* apartment, suggest that if you pretend you are somebody else, the grief will go away. Now it is certainly true that this period does promise a return of a measure of freedom and a return to self-interest, but what one does with it is entirely another matter. The Danish philosopher Sören Kierkegaard is quoted as saying that freedom was possibility and anxiety the possibility of freedom. In the empty-nest stage, anxiety emanates partly from the separation of children and partly from the challenge this brings for one's own development. However, an even more poignant source of anxiety is the awareness that can come with the empty nest that there is also an empty marriage. Finally, there is the greatest anxiety of all: with the children leaving home, one becomes aware of one's own death getting closer.

The separation of children from the family home creates both a physical space and a psychic space, a space that can expose not only what has gone, but what also was never there. The presence of children in a relationship can fill the space that lies between husband and wife, fill it with parental activity so that the intimacy that is missing is not seen or felt until the space is exposed by the children leaving. For many couples, getting into their fifties brings the additional loss of an emotional, nurturing and sustaining intimacy. This empty space can feel very threatening, particularly for women, as much of their identity can be tied up with being a mother. When this is added to loss of youth and an ageing and menopausal body, along with a partner who seems both distant and unsatisfactory, then it becomes immediately apparent why grief and depression are not uncommon reactions. It is far too simple to attribute the depression to hormonal changes—this is medical fantasy. What is actually going on is a profound shift, one which rocks the foundations of a woman's identity. It is the separation phase of the rite of passage from youth, and the task is to grapple with the losses, understand and allow for the sadness and avoid being labelled as simply "going through the Change". So often the pressure is to speak only of the positives of children leaving home, to keep up a good face to the world and to go along with the deception that loss is not actually occurring. Often the only person a woman can share her loss and confusion with is her GP, but his training and his own anxiety may lead him to medicalise it and prescribe a drug. The over-prescription of tranquillisers, while suiting the huge pharmaceutical companies and their often unwitting allies in the medical profession, is the price we pay for pretending that loss is not valid and that grief is not a healthy response. The real threat to ageing women is a complex set of social prejudices towards them as symbols of change, reinforced by rampant sexism and the fear of loss and death. Like the men who rush to buy Viagra, we collectively sanction technical, chemical and outward solutions to our losses, hoping they will just go away, rather than exploring them, reflecting on them, sharing them and seeing them as part of a process of renewal.

This medicalisation of the natural process of ageing connects to grief in another way. The simplest possible paradigm of the five stages of grief is denial, anger, bargaining, depression and finally acceptance. Choosing to take medication deals with four of the five "symptoms". It allows the temporary denial of ageing and loss, it controls the anger, masks the depression and permits us to make a child-like bargain with ourselves that the tablet, whilst not the solution, will ease the pain, a pain we fear we cannot bear. But the end result of this choice to medicalise can be the abortion of mourning itself and the cessation of growth and renewal. The empty nest becomes an empty womb when in fact the space can be, and indeed is, a fertile space waiting to receive a new conception of the self.

If a woman can bear the temporary barrenness and wait through the loss, then her mind and heart can begin, after years of nurturing others, to turn towards nurturing herself. This is how the space can become a fertile one. To put it another way, I would say that the empty nest, and all that goes with it, allows for a substantial shift, from a false sense of self to a true sense of self. Until this time, regardless of whether she has been engaged in the workforce or not, a woman has often been defined in relation to somebody else—as somebody's daughter, somebody's partner, somebody's mother, somebody's wife. The challenge of the empty nest is to be somebody in her own right. This shift, and both the difficulties and joys in it, was the most dominant theme to emerge in my interviews with women in their fifties. Whilst I had expected the empty nest to be an issue for these women, I had not fully anticipated how profound and how central it was to the search for self.

The empty-nest stage, then, like the awareness of

death which usually accompanies it, is the beginning of a gradual change whereby the pendulum of the psyche shifts from body to soul, from outer to inner and from a false self to a true self. It is the phase that enables a woman to hear the heroine's call to leave the familiar, to separate from the known and begin the task of moving through the psychic landscape to discover the self and ultimately to prepare for a conscious death. This need not be morbid or depressing, since it is not a change from life to death, but a change in life and part of the cycle of birth, life and death.

I have mentioned in passing several times the shift from a false to a true self, a process which I believe belongs properly in the middle phase of the rite of passage through the fifties. However, it is clearly necessary to discuss it in some detail at this point because it is such a vital idea for exploring the change a woman experiences at the empty-nest stage of marriage and family life. This shift or transmutation occurs in the space provided by the empty nest and the cessation of menstrual periods. This is also a space that can be filled and cluttered with irrelevancies and neurotic concerns about security, safety and the future. What sort of space it becomes, one that is cluttered and filled up, or one in which growth is conceived, depends partly on whether a woman has always maintained some sort of knowledge about this other, usually secret, self throughout her adult life. It was the British psychoanalyst Donald Winnicott who first articulated the idea of a false and true self.[1]

His extensive experience as a paediatrician as well as psychoanalyst gave him the distinct advantage of observing human nature from the beginning, long before words, and as a result he leaves one with the feeling that his theories are forged out of experience, not drawn from the pure air of academic speculation.

Winnicott's false self is not false in the pejorative sense of fake or phony. The false self, according to Winnicott, is defined by its function, which he sees as being to hide the true self—a function which is achieved in the main by the individual complying to the demands of others, starting with the mother in infancy. Not wishing to pursue in depth the psychoanalytic roots of this idea, I will only say that Winnicott based his notion of the true self on what he termed the behaviour of a "good enough mother". This is a mother who reads and meets the infant's needs rather than demanding the infant read and meet the mother's needs. At the most basic level this provides the infant with not just the experience of having its needs met, but the validation of its capacity to exert influence in the world by its own spontaneous gestures. It takes little imagination to see that these earliest repeated experiences form the basis of a sense of self as being legitimate and effective. On the other hand, if the mother is not able to read and respond to the child's early gestures and needs, and instead substitutes her own needs and views, then the child has to comply in order to survive. Thus a compliant self is developed rather than a spontaneous self. In my psychotherapeutic work I have been repeatedly struck by the fact that women who are stuck in a false compliant self invariably report mothers who were preoccupied, if not obsessed, with what they refer to as "proper manners". Thus from infancy through childhood into adulthood the false, compliant self is driven by the need for both survival and approval, and it grows until the ego becomes completely identified with it and the person believes this is who he/she actually is. There is clearly a strong similarity between this idea of Winnicott's and Jung's concept of the persona. Both see the function of this structure in the psyche as adaptation to the demands of normal social interaction, and in particular the need for approval. However, Winnicott provides a richer, and in my view far more useful, account of the origins and functions of the false self. Certainly it is a more valuable concept for understanding certain aspects of the fifties transition.

Winnicott's false self derives from the impulse to fit in, to accommodate to others. It is a little bit like an overcoat that one puts on to protect one's true self from the cold ravages of rejection and possible annihilation. Because it is worn all the time, it feels like a second skin, so that one can come to believe it is genuinely oneself. But inauthenticity of the false self is revealed by overcompliance, the relative absence of genuine creativity (as opposed to creative mimicry), and a certain underlying restlessness which is often accompanied by lapses in concentration and an overriding need to seek approval. If one could enter the mind of the person dominated by a false self, one would hear a thought process something like this: "I would really like to do this or that, but [and the *but* is underlined] what would my husband [or any other significant person] think of it?" The *but* is the moment of undoing, since it usually results in doubt and loss of enthusiasm for the idea because disapproval is anticipated. When this pattern is placed alongside what I see as the common desire in women to accommodate and facilitate things, it is not surprising that marriage and family life can cost women their sense of self. In a more cynical mood one might suggest that marriage is a form of institutional neurosis for some women, and not entirely beneficial for their psychic health. This is not, I should hasten to add, meant to imply that it does not meet many of their needs, such as a need for physical closeness, companionship, protection, but I believe that the cost of meeting these needs can be an undue level of compliance and accommodation that reinforces the false self. I should also add that the false self has a normal healthy level of functioning that enables us to fit into society. It allows for the achievement of compromise between one's individual needs and the needs of others. But if compromise becomes a form of habitual giving in at the ongoing expense of the true self, then the false self becomes a major psychological barrier to development.

The movement towards a true self is akin to what Jung termed the individuation process, and it continues throughout our lifetime. I think it reaches a crucial point at or around fifty—almost being the last substantial chance to make the shift in such a manner that it will enable us to die consciously. In fact the fifties transition is in my view the critical one in meeting the challenge of finding or uncovering the true self, a challenge that is undoubtedly present at each of the other major transitional points such as adolescence and mid-life. In adolescence we can clearly see the struggle, often expressed rebelliously and defiantly, to find some aspect of the true self. The disturbances of mid-life reveal a disillusion with and shedding of some false self aspects and the opening up of more space for the true self. But at both these stages there are still many outer demands to comply with—the need to survive financially, for example, career demands, family responsibilities. Hence the defiance of adolescence and sometimes of mid-life can be an overreaction to these demands rather than a genuine expression of the true self.

But by fifty one freedom that does emerge, at least as a possibility, is a lessening of the need for approval and the availability of opportunities to pursue activities that have for long been avoided. The pursuit of these activities can be an expression of the true self emerging from behind the protective wall of the compliant false self. As Germaine Greer, in her inimitable style, says of women at this stage,

> The middle aged woman may declare a taste for her own tipple, and for the first time a bottle of her own appears

on the drinks tray. She may become interested in betting on horses or playing bingo. She might even decide to change her house for a smaller one, or for a house in the country, or for a house that demands less housework and more gardening. She might even decide after years of putting up with him for the children's sake to divorce her husband. Whatever she decides the younger generation will click its collective tongue.[2]

Whilst much of this is tongue-in-cheek and goes close to trivialising the process, she nevertheless captures here the desire to change, characteristic of a woman of fifty-plus. But Greer of course has observed all this from outside the constraints of marriage and family life, and mainly from an intellectual position. Within marriage many subtle forces act against these legitimate desires for change and a movement towards a more direct experience of self. Not the least of these forces is the woman's need for approval from her husband and her fear of his rejection. This is particularly strong in long-standing marriages, which many are by the time a woman turns fifty. Habitual patterns of the interaction, often laid down when the wife was a young woman in her early twenties, are reinforced over the years of rearing children, which often leave her in a very dependent position with few options other than compliance. Karen Horney, an American psychoanalyst, echoes this point when discussing how men define women's experience. She says,

An additional and very important factor in the situation is that women have adapted themselves to the wishes of men and felt as if their adaptation were their true nature. That is, they see or saw themselves in the way that their men's wishes demanded of them; unconsciously they yielded to the suggestion of masculine thought.[3]

But at the empty-nest stage this state of affairs is at least open to question, since the external pressures to comply are substantially less. Julie, a woman in her late fifties, demonstrated both considerable courage and integrity as she arrived at a realisation that after over thirty years of marriage to a successful businessman husband, three children and a life that was materially very comfortable, she had to separate if she were to survive. This survival was both physically and psychologically necessary in her case, since she had developed a heart condition at fifty that was strongly resistant to treatment. At the same time she was struggling to give recognition and validation to her creative talents, which had been tangentially recognised by her whilst she remained within the confines of an orthodox middle-class marriage and an equally orthodox and restrictive middle-class family. Such families of origin can be the bastion of false selves. Indeed some members of the orthodox middle class have made an art form of the false self, cultivated around pseudo-élite social groups and reinforced at the regular ritual of the dinner party. "Niceness" in these circles replaces genuineness, and honesty is buried under pretension. This was the world that Julie had lived in from childhood; she had married a man who completely believed in it and had mixed with friends who supported it. But there was an artistic self, a self that had been rejected and disapproved of by her father in her teenage years, but that somehow managed to stay alive and breathe beneath the layers of niceness that surrounded her. She managed to cultivate her creative work to some extent through the marriage, although she rather took on her husband's dismissive view of it as just "her thing"—not something central to her being, but a little hobby on the side. By the time she was fifty, the space of the empty nest, the awareness of ageing, and the shortness of life itself had found their urgent expression first in her heart condition and then in her full and painful realisation that the marriage had only ever met her material needs and never her emotional needs. In fact it had only ever met and engaged her false self, but her dreams literally kept depicting a darker aspect which was forever beckoning her and at times even threatening to engulf her. She, like many women, had maintained an awareness of an inner, other self throughout the years of the marriage.

She recalled one memorable night as a turning point when the full awareness of her grief amidst the concern about her deteriorating heart condition hit her. She realised then that her husband was simply unavailable to her, a truth she had at some level always known but chosen not to know. In the terror of that night, full of suicidal thoughts, she had a "visit" from her grandmother, long since dead. This grandmother was a figure whom Julie had admired because of her capacity to do her own thing. On that night, as a result of the "visit", Julie began the task of embracing her true self and subsequently left the marriage, amidst much acrimony and power plays regarding money on her husband's part.

Plagued by doubts, she nevertheless slowly accepted the challenge of giving full expression to her creative life. Her heart condition improved dramatically, not through medical treatment, but because in separating from an unsustaining and un-nurturing marriage she had in fact treated the true self and listened to her heart. Her profound sadness on the night she realised she had to separate was only in part, and then only a small part, due to the loss of the marriage. In my view it was a far deeper grief than this: she was grieving for the past abandonment of her true self, a loss that literally could have killed her. This is a grief that I have observed in many people undergoing therapy, a moment when they first glimpse the profundity of the loss of relationship to the true self . . . it is literally a shocking, sad moment that can generate despair and remorse. It is also, though, a moment that elicits the possibility of self-reparation and renewal. Julie's life from fifty on is a testament to these truths and reinforces another point made by Winnicott in reference to the true self. That is, he considers the true self to be the source of creative life, since a person who listens to his or her true self is both spontaneous and has a well-developed capacity for using symbols. This was certainly true of Julie.

Marita is another person who heard the call of the true self at the empty-nest phase. She described always having a sense of another self that she referred to as a "sacrosanct self", but having pushed it under, hidden it, instead concentrating on being competent in the outer world. At fifty, she had a powerful archetypal dream that literally initiated her into her true self. She undertook therapy at this time with a male therapist who was able to respond to and accept the murmurings of the true self. After three years of therapy she felt her sacrosanct self had come to the fore and that the therapeutic process had been "transformative". The marriage had been a vehicle or container for the false self, the accommodating, obliging, competent self, and the renewed contact with her true self revealed a person who could not tolerate the constraints of being somebody she no longer felt she was. As part of her change in direction from outer to inner, since the false self had been exclusively outer, she visited the historic homeland of her ancestors, a trip that reaffirmed the source and took her back to the roots of her recently experienced true self. She changed jobs, separated from her husband, began working for herself, changed her Christian name to reflect her origins, and at the time of the interview was planning to move house. The internal change necessitates the outer. A renewed sense of self demands a new situation that reflects the change. It is not at all uncommon to find women changing their names as a result of re-connection to an aspect of the true self; sometimes a return to the maiden name following separation, other times a change of Christian name reflecting some important connection in their lives, one that recognises the lost aspects of themselves. For Marita, as for Julie, the process of reclaiming the self was accompanied by grief and physical symptoms—in her case a non-malignant breast cancer. The body very often expresses loss, as we know from studies of grieving, and both these women's physical complaints revealed the pain of their loss.

I want to briefly mention two other women because they also express the compelling urge to return to a sense of self long lost in marriage, and it was in both cases a return that occurred after adult children had left home. What these two women have in common is that, at least at the time I met them, they had not found it necessary to leave their husbands in order to express the true self. One woman in her early fifties had at previous times in her life experienced periods of depression. Coming into her fifties she was aware of feeling depressed again and was able to speak about her acute and overwhelming desire to be heard, to be heard and known by another. This was an experience that she had not had with her husband, despite the outer appearance of a stable and satisfying marriage. She described a lifetime of suppressed feelings which she had decided it was time to express. She, like the other women, had always had an awareness of another self, a self which she had shelved in the interests of motherhood, security and marital stability, a self that she had managed to keep secret from the world. The empty nest had removed one powerful constraint, children, and she seized the opportunity to use the space. She met another man, commenced a secret affair and for the first time felt heard. She declared she would be happy to die now as a result of experiencing the relationship. I would not consider this affair to be primarily a sexual acting-out aimed at retaining the illusion of youth such as is common in mid-life. On the contrary, it was enabling her to come alive and be true to her own experience and feelings; at least for the time being, Eros had prevented her from falling into the dark, depressive arms of Thanatos. Just as Marita had been initiated into herself via dream and Julie via her heart condition, this woman had been initiated into her long-suppressed self by a sexual affair. It was a choice of life over death, and hence at this time her confrontation with ageing and death was not yet really on the horizon—she had to first find life. As to the future of her marriage, it is difficult to predict, but like many women she declared that if finding herself through this relationship and being heard meant the marriage of thirty-plus years had to go, then so be it. This was not said in a cold, uncaring manner, it was simply the truth, a truth that many women have verbalised.

The last woman I want to mention was fifty-six at the

time I had my discussions with her. She revealed a history of always knowing about what she termed "the spark of self". As an older teenager she had travelled through Asia by herself in the late 1950s and early 1960s. This was a reasonably unusual and individualistic thing for a single female to do at that time. In her mid-thirties she undertook re-training and at fifty again returned to study, a study that this time involved overseas travel. She had managed to sustain this "spark of self" throughout what appeared to be a workable marriage. In her forties, when her husband wanted to change jobs and live in another state, she refused to go, having made several major compromises early in the marriage, and although her decision caused some marital conflict, she stuck by it. This was a case of listening to her "spark of self". Here refusal to compromise did not reflect rigidity but rather indicated that her awareness of the true self was strong enough to override the compliant self that had been instrumental in enabling the relationship to survive. The empty nest was for this woman merely a continuation of moments she had already known, and her choice to return to study involving periods overseas simply reflected her well-developed capacity to respect the true self, her "spark". She chose this over opting for her husband's approval, which could potentially have extinguished the spark. In her case, the marriage could absorb the change, and she did not have to separate from her husband. I did not meet him but I was left with the impression that he had his own struggles, was aware of them, and was open and reasonably sensitive to both himself and his wife. This is not always the case—the empty-nest phase can be very problematic for some husbands.

As I already mentioned, the empty nest impinges more on a woman's struggle to find herself than a man's. It is probably accurate to say that the male version of the empty-nest "syndrome" comes when a man is made redundant or retires from full-time work. It is in work that he secures and forms his identity, and as we will see later, the loss of it is as profound for him as the empty nest is for a woman. In men, whose natural disposition is to be more overtly aggressive than women, defiant and belligerent behaviours rather than compliance are the preferred option for protecting the true self and the feelings associated with it. So when a man is asserting himself right and left and belligerently refusing requests to do this or that, he is in fact very often expressing a false self, a version of self that society reinforces as masculine. It is often a protection against a softer, vulnerable, feeling self that he is afraid will be rejected if it is expressed. This is a result of his masculine social-isation.

The empty-nest stage for a man can reinforce this defiant false self as he struggles with his wife's changes. Marriage, or indeed any relationship, is a homeostatic system: you alter one part and it affects the other parts. A woman's decision to embrace aspects of her true self can, as we have seen, upset this homeostatic arrangement.

(Mind you, it is very often in need of disturbance!) For men insecure in their own identity, an emerging autonomy in their wives can threaten a loss of control. For many men the pattern of dominance and submission, rather than a mutual and equal engagement of opposites, is their notion of a good relationship. Hence a man's reaction to his wife's desire to pursue new interests and activities can be obstruction and objection. In many cases a history of the marriage would reveal this exact same pattern around the mid-life period. But at fifty, and with no dependent children, his wife becomes more difficult to control than when she was in her mid-thirties and engaged in full-time mothering. At a certain level of his psyche the children leaving home can remind him of his age and can reawaken memories of times past and opportunities foregone. Hence resentment of their freedom can build up towards the children and the wife, a resentment often fuelled by envy. He now can find himself with no one dependent on him, and, even more frightening, he can glimpse his own need for dependence. This, coupled with the need to control, can sometimes lead to him separating from his wife and marrying a younger woman. Whilst this choice is partly driven by an attempt to reassure himself of his sexual potency, it also stems from the desire to have control and to have somebody dependent upon him.

A man may also choose to defend against the anxiety generated by his wife's changes by deriding and denigrating her activities. Given a woman's need for male approval, this can seriously threaten her development and in some cases force a return to the false compliant self. He will be relieved by this, a pseudo-harmony will result and ultimately her life will go on unchanged, without awareness, and inevitably heading towards stagnation.

If, on the other hand, a man can accept and struggle with the anxiety generated by changes in his partner, then the result can be the opposite of stagnation. His acceptance of the necessity for his wife to change can engender in her a renewal of love, a renewal that can bring a revitalised connection to each other. When the need for change and growth is accepted by their partners, women feel valued, and the flow-on from this is often a renewal of sexual life. In the terms that we have been discussing throughout this book, the acceptance of change brings Eros into ascendance since a woman feels connected not only to herself but to her partner. Without the reconnection, Thanatos is in the ascendant and a diminution in sexual life and meaningful intimate contact is the inevitable result. Physical sickness can also emerge and instead of the fifties being a vital rite of passage into a more direct experience of self, it becomes a falling into age and despair.

To reiterate an earlier point, the critical step to be taken is the separation from old views of ourselves as men or women. For the man, this means separation from the view of himself as powerful, strong, decisive and in control. Rarely is he capable of this without outside promptings. At the empty-nest stage it is often the prompting of his wife that provides him with the first opportunity for his own growth. If he can grasp this opportunity and separate off from a traditional male view of himself, then he at the same time prepares himself for the more difficult change of retirement and the necessary shift in identity it brings. If he cannot grasp the nettle at the empty-nest stage and waits until retirement, it may well be too late, and he may find that his wife has made other psychological, if not physical, arrangements.

One man was able to share the difficulties accompanying the changes that took place in his marriage and family life at the empty-nest phase and then the subsequent exploration of the meaning they held for his own life. Bill had been married for over thirty years and had not long turned fifty when his life turned upside-down. At the time he held a senior administrative position in a large organisation, and his life was completely filled up with the demands of his job. His external personal life was typified by stability—a stable and warm marriage, a loving relationship with his two sons, plus the stability of living in the same house for a prolonged period. He and his wife were of similar age. By the time they turned fifty, both sons had left home and his wife felt an urgent need to change her life, to seize the opportunity for renewal and freedom that came with the empty nest. At her instigation, they sold the family home and bought a brand-new apartment in a trendy area of the city. On his own admission he was too busy to give any serious thought to the move, he just felt that if that was what his wife wanted then he would go along with it. Shortly after moving he became seriously depressed, and had to take the best part of a year off from his high-powered and responsible position. Depression was a complete shock to him, for he had never experienced such a profound sense of powerlessness and vulnerability. Throughout his adult life Bill had always regarded himself as an optimistic person who fully believed in the philosophy that mind can triumph over matter. His view had been that mental problems were basically of one's own making and could be overcome by sheer willpower. But he now found himself paralysed in the grip of Thanatos. One might well call this a breakdown but I prefer to call it a breakthrough, for after decades of suppression, his rich inner life had forced its way through. The loss of the family home was the focus of his conscious grief, a grief that did not completely make sense to him. But of course the home symbolised the predictable, orderly system that allowed him to avoid the demands and the needs of his feeling life. The anger that is part of grief found its expression in criticisms and regrets about moving to the new apartment. There was nothing about it that he could find acceptable. The extent of his unhappiness caused them to sell the apartment and return to accommodation in the area they had originally lived in. One is left to wonder how his wife might have felt about this and whether it was a return to an old, pre-empty-nest, accommodating behaviour on her part. However, it may well be that it was a compromise that she made in the interests of the marriage surviving and out of her concern for the mental well-being of her partner.

For Bill, with the assistance of therapy, this was the beginning of a major period of self-reflection. He struggled with the variability of his moods, with fluctuations in his hopes that it would all pass and he would simply go back to work. Months passed, and increasingly he was able to make sense of his so-called breakdown through the exploration of the meaning of his rich dreams. He connected to profound feelings of loss back in childhood, the loss of his own feeling and spontaneous life in adulthood as he climbed, or was pushed, up the corporate ladder, and also the sadness he had felt at his children leaving home. The loss of his home symbolised these additional losses and literally woke him up, or initiated him, into his inner life. Over time, acceptance of his feeling life grew, together with an awareness of how it had been sacrificed. He finally returned to work with a very different sense of time and urgency, such a different sense that he reached a point where the job had no meaning for him and he took an early retirement. He said that he now found himself with "a sense that I need to rekindle a future life which has the same pulling power as looking forward did when I was twenty. A period of active waiting and hope, power and choice". He had, via the disturbance brought on by his wife's desire to "rekindle" her life, found part of himself. Thus for this man the empty nest was a painful but highly creative period. Fortunately for him, he had a partner who was able to respond to her own inner world, even if her original choice of expression for it was perhaps a little premature. The urge to change houses at fifty-plus is determined not just by the obvious fact of a house being too big following the children's departure, it is also a significant expression of the need to re-locate one's self. Where we live is a symbolic expression of where we live in ourselves. Hence changes to where we live in ourselves often demand changes in where we live physically. The only risk is that we will change houses in the hope that it will change where we live in ourselves. This may well have been the situation with Bill's wife, but in the long run she had sufficient maturity to reflect upon and learn from the experience. It would have been far more destructive to have not made the choice to move, because Bill's wife would have remained stuck in her old definition of herself and probably become angry and resentful. He, on the other hand, would have gone on as busy and important as ever and not discovered what a rich, imaginative and feeling side he had. Certainly there were times when he felt no hope for himself, or the future, but that was the separating phase of his initiation and subsequent beginning of a renewal. The breakdown-cum-breakthrough gave him the opportunity to let go and grieve as a necessary prelude to change. But Bill is not the rule, regrettably, he is an exception. The more characteristic response of men is to exert control and to override their feelings with will and ego.

———————

1   D. Winnicott, "Ego Distortion in terms of True and False Self" in *The Maturational Processes and The Facilitating Environment*, Karnac Books, London 1990, pp. 140–52.
2   G. Greer, op.cit., p. 57.
3   K. Horney, *Feminine Psychology*, ed. H. Kelman, Routledge & Kegan Paul, London, 1967, pp. 56–7.

5

Androgyny in the Fifties

A most significant area of the fifties experience, one that comes into full view at the empty-nest phase, is the question of identity, specifically sexual identity and sexual roles. We have seen that body influences identity, so too does the biological reality that we contain both male and female genes affect an individual's sexual identity. The psyche always has a biological sub-stratum; conversely, the reality of male and female genes finds its parallel at the psychic level, in the existence of what has been termed the masculine and feminine principles.

The idea of masculine and feminine being inherent in human nature is of course a very ancient one that finds clear exposition in the Chinese philosophy of yin and yang. The Chinese considered yin and yang to be the primal polarity not only in the individual but also in the cosmos, and it constitutes a vital part of the practice of Chinese medicine. The yin, or feminine principle, includes such qualities as space, continuity, nourishing, purposelessness, unity, and acausal perception. Yang, the masculine principle, includes time, individualisation, differentiation, order, purpose and linear causal thinking.

We have already discussed these attitudes in passing, but it is necessary to return to them and explore them again. David Gutmann, who has written comprehensively and insightfully on the theme of psychoanalysis and ageing, has empirically demonstrated, using anthropological evidence, that there is a psychological move towards androgyny in both men and women in many cultures.[1] His evidence mainly refers to men, indicating that as a man gets older he experiences a re-emergence of feminine attributes. In old age proper, seventy-plus, not only his demeanour but also his body changes, in an increasingly feminine direction. Likewise for women, in the post-parental period there is a psychological move towards increased masculine attributes and orientation. Indeed, some older women at first glance appear to be men. The voice deepens, the posture changes and in some cases the woman appears to over-identify with the emergence of masculinity in both her dress and general demeanour. This over-identification with the masculine polarity is often at the expense of the feminine and is very different from integration. Her older husband or partner can at the same time exhibit a growing interest in domesticity, and in the extreme become over-identified with his feminine side by being fussy and obsessive. An older man's stooped posture often reflects timidity and a fearfulness of being in the world, a stance that many women, at different stages in their life, can identify with. In the elderly, we can clearly observe the physical emergence of opposite sex qualities, but it has begun long before. It is by focusing on the earlier emergence that we can appreciate the psychological meaning of this seemingly natural movement towards androgyny as we get older. We also have to take into account an overlapping factor, and that is the re-emergence of narcissism in both genders. The empty-nest phase, as we have seen with some of the women we have discussed, brings with it a retrieval of a measure of narcissism which is not pathological, but rather signifies a return of healthy interest in the self, after the pressing demands of children.

It is this absence of parental responsibility in association with ageing that evokes the move towards androgyny. The task of parenting, even if a woman is working full-time, generally brings with it a parcelling out of psychological and physical labour along gender lines. Socially directed pressures to change the traditional division of labour have managed, in the main, only to change outer behaviour and even then minimally, within the domain of family life. In the psyche, men still seem to take on the traditional male role, reflecting the masculine principle or yang quality, of being out in the world, giving form, taking action and providing for dependants. Women, on the other hand, nowadays add a sizeable proportion of the male role to the existing female roles, which express such qualities as nurturance, receptiveness, connectedness and openness to the feeling life. The end result of this division of psychological labour is that throughout the active parental years, each partner concedes to the other aspects of their own sexual bimodality, in the interests of fulfilling the parental tasks. This period, which nowadays is increasingly prolonged due to adult children staying longer in the parental home, also demands self-abnegation, or at least modification of each parent's narcissism or self-interest. Indeed, one of the fundamental maturing experiences of being a parent is just this, that both sexes have to learn to modify and delay their own needs in the interests of the child. Undoubtedly this can happen in any caring relationship, whether that be with an individual partner or through some form of caring work, but being a parent is perhaps the most obvious and immediately available reason for modifying narcissism. Indeed, David Gutmann states, "Childless women have never experienced that great transformation of narcissism which renders the child's life more precious than their own".[2]

Whilst fathers do not have the potent experience of giving birth to a child and feeding it, the task of protecting, rearing and loving one's child does on many occasions demand a foregoing of one's own needs.

To return to the empty nest: the child leaving means that the demands for the parental division of labour wane, there is a less compelling rationale to maintain it along gender lines, and there begins what one would technically term "a return of the repressed" in both genders. Men begin, sometimes reluctantly, to make contact with their femininity, women with their masculinity, and both genders with their earlier repressed narcissistic or self-interested needs. The end result can be marital turmoil and considerable confusion and uncertainty after years of living in a structure that worked. This structure is disturbed and often dismantled. The previous examples of women who reclaimed a sense of self and moved away from an accommodating false self clearly illustrate the conflictual marital patterns that can emerge at this stage.

David Gutmann's work on androgyny confirms thoughts that Jung put forward some seventy years ago. In fact it is to Jung then we will temporarily return, since his theory allows for an insightful look at this androgynous move in the empty-nest phase of marriage. Jung termed the masculine principle within a woman the "animus" and the feminine within a man the "anima".[3] It might be useful to discuss their meaning a little further so that we can see them in their own right as archetypal energies. The animus is a male image in a woman's unconscious, usually clearly visible in dreams, that symbolises the attributes of organisation, order, logic and form, whereas the feminine image in a man's psyche symbolises feeling, receptiveness, nurturance and connectedness. Both these figures, according to Jung, have like any archetype a positive and negative face.

The abovementioned qualities are the positive faces, the negative being in the case of the animus, rigidity, power, dominance, an obsessional need for order and opinionated attitudes. For the anima, the negative attributes would include moodiness, petulance, smothering, aimlessness and obsequious behaviour. The relationship between these archetypal attributes or energies and marriage is that we tend to unconsciously choose a partner who reflects our own opposite. So in addition to the overt, physical and visible person we partner, we also partner our opposite inner qualities, or respectively anima or animus. This, if you like, is the unconscious marriage whilst the one we legalise is the conscious one.

The psychological function of this arrangement is that our partners tend to contain, via projection, our split-off and unacknowledged opposite gender attributes. This forms the unconscious base upon which the division of psychological labour is built during the parenting years. The first glimpse we receive of their existence is usually a marital quarrel. Such quarrels reveal the truth of the assertion that "anima" and "animus" together leads to animosity! So a man can become petulant and moody and his female partner opinionated and rigidly logical, all culminating in misunderstanding since the argument is not about what it ostensibly appears to be, but really about anima and animus. Apart from these sort of quarrels, it is at mid-life that the first substantial contact is made with the contra-sexual elements within us. So mid-life is usually about anima or feeling issues for men and often, although less so in our modern times, about animus or being-in-the-world issues for women. But the outer demands of parenthood at mid-life tend to lead to a repression of opposite qualities. Alternatively they can be sexualised and acted out but not integrated, by one partner seeking the anima or animus in relationships outside the marriage.

With the departure of children, the sexual bimodality returns unencumbered by outer constraints. It is now apparent that the animus is the power behind a woman's choice to abandon her false self at this stage and literally give form and organisation to her true self so it can be in the world. The emergence of the masculine principle allows her to begin to take control of her life and to feel an increased sense of autonomy. Hence many women speak of feeling so much energy and well-being around fifty-five. The lifting of parenting constraints leads a woman to feel entitled to pursue her own interest and re-invest in her self. How well she has dealt with her mid-life transition will to a large extent determine how effectively she expresses this later move toward androgyny in her fifties. If she chooses to ignore or deny it at mid-life, then there is a fair chance she will continue the same strategy in her fifties. These tend to be women who are frightened of their own aggression, fearing that it will in some manner render them less feminine and therefore less desirable to men, and thus ultimately place their dependence on men in jeopardy.

They tend to live out their masculine part by continuing to project it onto their husbands, just when some of the men need to develop the more passive, receptive feminine side. Because the wives' projections inhibit their husbands' access to femine qualities, the result can, in the long run, be disappointing relationships characterised by bitter mutual recrimination. An inability to allow for and accept masculine attributes, now clearly available in the fifties, leaves a woman impoverished and with a sense of having lost control of her own destiny, feelings which can only exacerbate the problems of age. This repression of the masculine energy commonly finds an unhealthy expression in physical complaints as a sense of despair and futility creeps in. The move into androgyny is critical, since it forms a psychological preparation for the later stage of old age, dependency and ultimately death without falling into despair. The integration of masculine energy gives a woman a renewed zest and the desire to be part of life instead of being a helpless victim.

The emergence of the masculine principle at fifty can also awaken in some women a desire for homo-erotic relationships—it is not unusual to find this theme in women's dreams around this stage. Some will choose to sexualise the homo-erotic desires and enter into a lesbian relationship, either permanent or temporary, at this time. This is a clear expression of the emergence of the masculine principle in their psyche, a principle that may well have always had a strong presence, but was perhaps repressed in the interest of others. For other women it simply leads to an even stronger desire for female friendship which does not involve a sexual relationship, but nevertheless one which affords an opportunity for both assertion and emotional intimacy and freedom from a stereotyped female role.

Within marriage, a woman experiencing her androgynous qualities can become more active sexually, less inhibited and more inclined to take the initiative than in the past. She can delight in the knowledge of being free of any possibility of pregnancy, feel the freedom of no children around, and also feel the pulse of wanting to express a new-found sense of self. Fuelled by anxiety at the loss of youth and by the desire to shed a false sense of self, the emergence of masculine energy can empower a woman to pursue extramarital relationships. In fact, some marriages are possibly sustained by an unconscious or tacit agreement around this choice. Such an arrangement, if both parties are in agreement, can help to maintain the erotic energy within the marriage itself. In the world, the re-emergence of repressed masculine aspects can also provide a woman with a renewed sense of purpose, so she may choose to change her employment and not uncommonly to shift from being an employee to being self-employed. Behind these moves is the hand of the positive animus. As we saw with Bill's wife in the previous section, it was the energy behind her desiring a change of both lifestyle and home.

Karen, who was fifty-four at the time of our interview,

is a fine example of a woman who first made productive contact with her masculine aspects at mid-life and then was able to give even fuller expression to them in her early fifties. At mid-life she left an unsatisfactory marriage, or perhaps more accurately an unsatisfying one that simply did not meet her emotional needs, despite the apparent pleasantness of the relationship. In passing one could say this of many seemingly "pleasant" marriages, that the cost of pleasantness is a repression of feeling and passion and real communication. They are marriages in which the spouses' unconscious connection to each other has often been repressed and hence there is no meaningful feeling connection. Karen, as a single mother, raised her own daughter, who is now in her mid-twenties. She described two things that had had a profound effect on her around the age of forty-nine: First, she became acutely aware of her own mortality, and second, seeking a male partner became of less importance to her, something she described as having driven her through her thirties and forties. At fifty, she left her paid employment and set up her own consultancy business. She recounted that she now felt a strong sense of herself and had a renewed vision for the future. This had so far expressed itself in a change of work and also a change of house. As if to underline the influence of Eros in this renewal, she also said that, somewhat ironically, in letting go the importance of seeking a male partner in the outer world she has observed that she was having far more sexual fantasies than previously. One could take this to mean first the presence of Eros in the renewal and second some integration of opposite genders within herself, the fantasy representing an inner, not outer, union of opposites. She felt that whereas previously her body had gone out to the world in particular to seek a male partner, it was now going into herself, giving her a renewed sense of autonomy and empowerment. What Karen's situation reveals is confirmation of both the re-emergence of the masculine, but more importantly her willingness to take risks at mid-life, to preserve her sense of self, which could only have full expression when she was free of the responsibilities of child rearing. She had in one sense allowed Thanatos to do his work, to disconnect from old definitions of herself as someone who needed a partner and as someone who sought the security of a regular wage. These disconnections were both painful and anxiety-provoking for her but had also made possible the renewal and availability to embrace the animus energy and recreate a new vision for her life.

Kathleen is fifty-six, a married woman and mother of three. She exhibits a pattern of having an acute awareness of her need to develop, but through the mid-life transition and the years of child-rearing she deferred it, partly out of consideration for others and commitment to her children, and more poignantly through grave self-doubts about her ability. Whilst trying several short-term courses through her thirties and forties she maintained a long-standing desire to be involved in helping others. As

she approached fifty she undertook personal therapy
with a male therapist who was able to mirror and reflect
back her own masculine side. This coincided with her
children becoming more independent, and she set about
instigating some realistic plans for re-education in the
counselling field. The lessening of parental responsibility
along with the insights gained in therapy coincided with
the emergence of her repressed masculine energy, and
she completed a course which gave her an increase in her
self-confidence and ability. By the time the children had
all left home she was poised to return to the world of
paid work, something she had not done since her early
twenties. Whilst she had foregone choice and risk-taking
at mid-life, she had nevertheless maintained a consciousness about herself and her own needs. The empty nest,
and a marriage that could satisfactorily absorb the
change although not without some disturbances,
provided the opportunity, and the re-emergence of
masculine energy provided the impetus. The end result
was a substantial movement toward her true self. The
fifties for Kathleen, whilst involving a noted sadness
about the loss of youth and the motherhood role which
had been very important to her, and also the perceived
loss of her physical attractiveness, had nevertheless seen
the development of her inner self. The losses coexisted
alongside the gains, but mostly the renewed sense of self
prevailed and the experience of rewarding work
sustained her.

There is an ever-increasing group of women who

develop animus qualities in the first half of life; for these women, the second half, including the fifties, can reveal the emergence of the feminine principle, or anima qualities. At fifty or so, these women, who are usually strongly career-oriented, experience the re-emergence of the feminine attributes, or yin qualities, that have often been suppressed in the interests of a career. It is therefore not uncommon to find successful career women approaching fifty deciding on a complete change, usually in the direction of increased simplicity, fewer demands and work done from home. For some this change represents a re-connection to the feminine part of themselves through choosing a new career in the helping professions. This is a move towards androgyny from the other direction.

For men, the post-parental emergence of androgyny can be a mixed blessing and again is shaped by the patterns of resolution at mid-life. For men coming into their fifties the re-emergence of their femininity alongside the female partner's reconnection to her masculinity can cause considerable angst. Until now he has usually projected his feminine self onto his wife, lover or some fantasised other woman, but rarely acknowledged it as part of himself. By the time he is in his fifties, these options are less available, and he can find himself staring full on at his feminine self. The realisation that so-called feminine traits are part of his own internal landscape and are not exclusive to his female partner can lead to panic and confusion. If, on the other hand, he has at mid-life made preliminary contact with his inner world he is far less likely to panic. I found in my interviews that the creative men were relatively untroubled and indeed often welcomed both the reawakening of the feminine and the changes in their marriage which freed them to pursue their creative talents in even greater depth. Such men have, throughout their adult lives and often acutely at mid-life, had some awareness of an inner life, a feminine aspect of their psyche. It is not new to them at fifty, since their creative work has usually involved the feminine principle and energy.

But men who have repressed this aspect of themselves often display a pattern of marrying women who have been willing to be submissive and live out for them the denied feminine aspect. When his wife emerges in the world with renewed autonomy, a man can experience this as her being dominating and accuse her of deliberately castrating him. What is behind this fear is the dread of discovering his own dependency and passivity. It is passivity that I believe frightens such a man most of all, awakening terror around feelings of vulnerability, loss of power, loss of potency and indecisiveness that he perceives as weakness. He does not experience the reappearance of the feminine in his psyche as positive, primarily because it has remained undeveloped, been ignored at mid-life, and usually remained inseparable from his infantile experiences of his mother. He thus will try to take flight from his discoveries, and perhaps seek a new relationship with a younger woman who he thinks will restore the status quo—i.e., be dependent and not threaten him with his own feminine side. If this option is not open to him, for whatever reasons, then another possibility is that his reawakened passive, dependent side will find its way into his body, where he will manifest any number of psychosomatic complaints. These can allow him to be dependent and vulnerable without separating from his own masculine identity—after all, he is not dependent in his own eyes, he is merely unwell.

Other men resort to the well-worn path of "When in doubt, take action" and defend against the emergence of femininity in their fifties by increasing their workload on the basis that moving targets are harder to hit. But what is going on in all these situations is a refusal to change and grow, a refusal to embrace the natural movement towards androgyny that comes with being in one's fifties. As I have said, I suspect that fear of passivity is central to this refusal because it is seen as unmasculine, but also perhaps because it awakens anxieties about homo-erotic feelings. Just as for women, the emergence of the feminine in men can evoke homo-erotic fantasies, which can be felt as a desire for closer relationships with other men—relationships that are not based on competitiveness but include nurturance, compassion and companionship. In some men homo-erotic fantasies are expressed in sexual form. However, such homosexuality often appears to have more to do with wanting to experience the self as female in relation to a male, being the receptive and not the active partner, than a literal attraction to men. If androgyny takes this path, it can create panic and shock and lead to marital breakups, although I think it is preferable to take time to explore its meaning fully before rushing into separation. Some couples may decide to integrate some form of bimodal sexuality within the confines of the marriage.

What the emergence of the contrasexual component also brings is an opportunity for the couple to adapt to the slow physical diminution of sexual drive by expanding their focus of sexual satisfaction. Instead of a sexual life being dominated by a genital focus, other means of meeting erotic needs can be developed and sexuality can become more diffuse. For example, the eroticism of skin can be included as part of achieving intimacy and as an alternative to the preoccupation with the penis and penetration. This in turn will facilitate a shift from the exclusivity of the phallus to the inclusivity of the body, something that is valuable in the wake of sadness at the loss of a youthful body.

A man who can accept his femininity is more likely to make these shifts, since he will allow himself to be a receiver, rather than always being the initiator and the one in control. Men not able to embrace the move towards androgyny are stuck with performance anxiety and fear of impotence. The feminine principle allows for a diffuseness of sexuality that can greatly enrich the intimacy of a relationship. But, as always, this movement demands that men separate from their stereotyped masculine view of themselves, face the unknown, allow the feelings to emerge and move towards a redefinition of what it might mean to be an older man moving into his sixties, where physical strength and potency are going to be more difficult to find and where the integration of masculine and feminine is the more phase-appropriate task.

By both parties acknowledging and understanding their androgynous nature, the empty-nest phase of marriage can be like the alembic vessel of the alchemist in which transformation can occur. In alchemy this is a transformation that first requires separation, the distillation and purification of the separated material, followed by the coming together of opposites in a symbolic form of gold and silver or sun and moon. The alchemist held that if the separation was not done properly then the end result was what they called a false *coniunctio*, a false marriage, in which all the material simply fused together and finished up a sticky mess that took them back to where they started. On the other hand, if the material was well separated then a true *coniunctio* or union, as opposed to fusion, occurred and out of this union of opposites the philosopher's stone, or philosophical gold, was born. So it is with marriage: a separation from fixed and familiar views of ourselves and the sorting out of various different components afford the necessary condition for a fruitful union. Failure to accept the inevitability of change, in this case the emergence of androgyny, results in a messy fusion in which partners have to sometimes resort to a pattern

of fighting, quarrelling and bickering in order to establish a more primitive form of separateness.

---

1   David L. Gutmann, "Psychoanalysis and Ageing: A Developmental
    View", in S.I. Greenspan and G.H. Pollock (eds), *The Course of Life:
    Psychoanalytic Contributions Toward Understanding Personality Development*,
    vol. III: *Adulthood and the Ageing Process*, National Institute of Medical
    Health, Washington, 1980, pp. 489–517.
2   ibid., p. 516.
3   C.G. Jung, "Anima and Animus", *Collected Works* vol. 7, Routledge
    & Kegan Paul, London, 1953, pp. 188–211.

6

The Grandparenting Phase: Renewal or Decay?

Before leaving the topic of marriage and family life, I want to discuss one other area, and that is grandparents. This is for many, if not most people, a deeply gratifying experience, bringing profound joy in the renewal of life along with an opportunity to re-live the pleasures of parenting without the full-time burden. It is parenthood with freedom. But the new life of the grandchild also heralds the life of the grandparents coming towards its end. It is the paradox of newness and beginnings highlighting oldness and ends. Thus the arrival of a grandchild is a potent reminder of the reality of time passing and time running out. For some women it can also be a means by which they avoid the empty nest and thereby avoid any meaningful confrontation with their own self. They hastily move from motherhood to grandmotherhood and pray that no space will enter in the meantime. Other women, while acknowledging the desire to have a grandchild and the joy of it, are able to also acknowledge the need for time between the ending of the active mothering years and the arrival of a grand-child. These are the women who perceive the space of the empty nest as a creative womb in which the self can be reborn. Those who welcome the rush into grand-parenting are literalising and projecting out this symbolic rebirth onto the physical world of the grand-child. It is doubtful whether concretisation of an inner process can lead to a continuing renewal of self.

But there is another generation of "grandparent", and that is one's own children's grandparents—the grand-parents who are one's own ageing parents. An ageing parent is a symbol not of renewal as a grandchild is, but of decline, decay and ultimately death. Many individuals in their fifties, having just got free of their children, are faced with the often child-like demands of ageing, dependent and frail parents. It is a striking fact of nature that both these experiences should often coincide and create such an awareness of the polarity of life and death.

In my view, ageing parents play a more significant role in stimulating people in their fifties to get on with their lives and development than do grandchildren. But this response is mostly forged out of fear and not neces-sarily out of a genuine desire to develop. At the root of this fear is the confrontation with one's own physical and mental deterioration that an aged and frail parent can evoke. Many people in their fifties find themselves first helping an aged parent, often a widowed one, to maintain a sense of independence, and then having to make decisions about full-time care. This can be a source of conflict among siblings as they struggle with their own individual agendas and issues regarding getting old, in particular the question of their own dependence and vulnerability. The outer image of an aged and deteriorating parent, a figure that was through our childhood big and powerful, is a very difficult experience to integrate. Inevitably it provokes a frightening glimpse of one's self twenty-five or thirty years on, and it is more often than not an unwelcome rather than reassuring glimpse. It is a glimpse of the biological truth of age, a picture of the end of the process that one is just becoming engaged with at fifty. One man discussed the shock he felt on realising that his much-admired father was actually losing his memory. He strongly identified with his father and this identification extended to seeing himself in a similar state twenty-five to thirty years hence. With such persistent anxiety and publicity about senility or Alzheimer's disease as there is nowadays, an ageing senile parent can truly be a frightening image of the future. It is also a powerful metaphor of the decay that age invariably brings. The loneliness of a widowed parent is another disturbing image that causes angst in the soul of many people at or around fifty. At this stage they often still have a partner themselves, but the widowed, dependent status of their parents activates the gravest of fears concerning their own future loneliness if they should find themselves widowed. Conversations and guesses amongst people in their fifties about "who will go first" can be humorous, but fear and anxiety is often not far away in these discussions.

In fact, this theme of independence and dependence that so often characterises discussions about aged parents is central to anxiety about one's own ageing. Being dependent on others is what many people fear about getting old, and it is a fear that starts to take hold in one's fifties. Obsessive preoccupation with superannuation can be a reflection of a deeper anxiety centring around dependency and old age. Being dependent on the care of others is a particularly frightening prospect for those individuals who have led a very self-sufficient existence, financially and emotionally. These are often people who did not have their own dependency needs met when they were young. Being sent to boarding school at an early age, having a mother who was depressed, or one who simply did not want a child, or alternatively a very large family with lots of siblings, might contribute to one's dependency needs not being met in childhood. The outcome of this can be a sort of counter-phobic response—the child becomes fiercely independent, in order to avoid ever putting himself or herself in a vulnerable situation again. Such people will sometimes find their way into careers that allow them to care for others, which is not in any way meant to imply that they do not do it adequately and with integrity. But what it does achieve, at an unconscious level, is a warding-off of their own anxieties about being dependent by projecting their dependency needs upon those that they are caring for. Motherhood and a very large family is another way of meeting a person's dependence needs via projection.

These sorts of responses prevent an understanding and acceptance of the fact that all human beings are dependent to some extent. People who fear the dependence that age brings don't distinguish between a disabling and destructive dependence that thwarts autonomy, and a healthy, enabling dependence that facilitates growth. For these people, old age and ageing parents in particular, confirms their worst fears and often reawakens some powerful feelings from childhood regarding dependency. These people cannot imagine that others might care for them willingly: they project their own fears into the future and see caring only as an obligatory behaviour that is not done with love or willingness. Such people often have had full-time careers and the thought of stopping full-time work can be a frightening one, since it crystallises anxiety around dependence. It is to the area of work in the fifties that we now turn.

7

Work and the Fifties

Like relationships, work is a major source of identity, for some women now almost as much as for men. Therefore it ought not be too surprising that work is centrally involved in the fifties transition. The issues around work do not conform to a simple straightforward pattern, but it is probably safe to say that by the mid-fifties little new is likely to arise in relation to one's work, other than the possibility of redundancy or early retirement. Many of the career goals set in midlife have either been reached, or it is painfully clear that they are not going to be achieved, at least to the level one might have hoped for at thirty-five. There seems to be a sort of plateauing effect, and regardless of the nature of one's work, a certain measure of repetition and boredom starts to creep in. In some respects it can feel like the mid-life transition again; however, there is neither the time nor the energy available at fifty-five to contemplate a major career change. Many people therefore arrive at a somewhat resigned acceptance of the status quo until retirement or redundancy and the collection of a pension.

In the current age we are witnessing many changes in the workplace, not the least of which is technological change. This is taking place within a changing work culture, driven by the ideology of corporate globalisation that by anyone's measure is not the slightest bit interested in the well-being of individuals. In my own professional practice over the past decade, I have been very conscious of a marked increase in stress generated from work, in particular among people working in organisations. Person after person will talk with despair of physical and psychological overload, the sheer sense of always being under pressure, never having enough time, and being buried under paper (a metaphor that has a certain chilling truth about it). They also invariably express distress concerning under-staffing and the refusal of organisations to replace employees who have left. Corporatisation and its sinister twin, marketing, have captured the individual and are holding the soul to ransom.

The problem has been exacerbated by technological change so that our capacity to generate information has far outstripped our ability to process it. We are emailed out (which we could well spell emaled rather femaled!). Organisational culture, through individual contracts and "downsizing", has created an environment which is dominated by profound uncertainty. Most people I have seen professionally are seriously affected psychologically by this culture of uncertainty, which generates fear and considerable anxiety regarding one's work performance and adequacy. Undoubtedly we need a measure of uncertainty to stimulate us to perform and learn, but there is clearly a limit to the amount we can bear before we are crippled by it. Low job security has the effect of pitting employee against employee, so that being in large organisations appears to have more in common with life in the jungle than with some form of work in a civilised society. Uncertainty evokes aggression and territoriality, which are jungle behaviours. Globalisation has weakened the sense of connection to each other, weakened empathy and compassion, and led to a disconnection from work itself. The new work culture has banished Eros and reduced connection to some trendy market-driven and consultant-contrived team-work exercise. This Eros vacuum has left a space in which Thanatos does its work through envy and a breakdown in sense of community. The banishing of Eros to the margins also leaves the possibility of it manifesting itself in the more perverse form of sexual harassment in the workplace. Yet financial necessity forces people to be captives of this uncivilised system.

People reaching their fifties have witnessed this cultural change, the erosion of what they once knew work to be. In short, they are in culture shock. When there is no meaningful connection to work, the result is an inner alienation and emptiness. Freud, when asked what were the requirements for human happiness, replied "to love well and work well". In our present Western society there is a great deal of unhappiness, much of which comes from meaningless, disconnected, over-demanding work and the absence of time for relationships.

One reaction to this inner alienation or emptiness is to to fill it up with material gains and if possible power. But by fifty-five or so, to be still pursuing these goals is to be denying the significance of ageing and the stage of life that one is in. Men of fifty-plus ought to be beginning a shift from power to mentoring, from dominance to influence, ego to self. However, there is a significant link here with the emergence of androgyny. If a man cannot tolerate and accept his feminine self, he is unlikely to accept and make this shift from power to mentoring. This is the shift that demands a change in values and the fundamental swing in the centre of his psychic gravity from outer to inner, from ego to self. It is a shift that can only be made by conscious acceptance of the feminine principle which makes it possible for him to be receptive and not preoccupied with action. The men and women who refuse to hear the call of the feminine at fifty are the very same people who cannot give up work, cannot accept slowing down, cannot give up power and cannot alter their priorities from material possessions to psychological and spiritual growth. The real threat that drives these workaholics is the fear of stopping and actually running into themselves. Retirement and redundancy is their version of the empty nest, so they fill it rather than allow for a creative renewing space. The reality of their own gradual decline and inevitable death does not occur to these workaholics, since their thinking is outer-directed and usually riddled with fantasies of omnipotence and immortality. They are desperate to show the world how successful they are and they fight ferociously to convince themselves of their own importance. Here the false self has been made into an art form, and the true self is a shrivelled carcass at the bottom of the psyche, buried beneath possessions. In their refusal to separate from their youth, and from youthful values, these people refuse the true heroic call to integrate and embrace more than the material world, and refuse at the same time to shift from outer values to inner ones, from body to soul.

What these people, more often men than women, have in common with another group of employees is an obsession with the Holy Grail of self-funded pensions. In Australia there are television advertisements espousing the joys of superannuation. Several people are interviewed in the advertisements, each sharing their fantasies of retirement, and fantasies they are indeed. They are composed of the usual collection of more time to play golf/travel/garden, etc., etc. The point is that with work becoming increasingly a disconnected experience and thereby increasingly meaningless, superannuation becomes an idealised fantasy of some blissful future time when all their meaninglessness will be behind them. Superannuation is like a secular heaven, a rewarding after-work life. It has therefore all the hallmarks of a sort of revived Calvinistic Protestantism, which suits the corporate mentality exceeding well since it negates individualism and difference.

In itself, a self-funded pension scheme is probably not a bad idea, but the fantasising about some paradisaical future state is a defence against loss and it is therefore not a helpful pattern. I have lost count of the number of people I have seen professionally who, while sharing considerable distress and unhappiness about their current work situation, say they cannot possibly take early retirement because they need to preserve their superannuation benefits. It doesn't seem to occur to them that the cost of their unhappiness and stress may well be an early death, for which superannuation will not be much use. Behind the superannuation fantasy of a perpetually blissful other world is another, subtler fantasy—that one is going to live a very long time.

Connected to these issues, and perhaps contributing to them, is the split we make between work and non-work. It is similar to the split we make between youth and age, dependence and independence, and male and female. A major developmental task coming into one's fifties is to begin to heal these splits and integrate the opposite.

This split and the alienation of many from their work are lesser issues to creative individuals. For such people the distinction between work and non-work is blurred and the question of retirement often irrelevant, since the only thing a self-employed creative person can retire from is themselves. Their work is not something they do, but something they are; it is an expression of the self. Despite the tremendous emotional strains creative work entails, and foregoing of material comforts and gains, it brings to most creative people an irreplaceable level of meaning. In a sense, the creative life is the antidote to work as most people experience it, since creative work transcends the inner alienation and disconnection so characteristic of modern non-creative work and heals the split between work and non-work.

Several creative people I interviewed expressed the view that retirement was irrelevant and that the only effect of ageing on their relationship to their work was to deepen the movement inwards rather than outwards, as they increasingly freed themselves from the outer demands of the ego and the need to prove their worth in the world. They all spoke warmly of this freedom. One writer's main reflection on getting into his fifties was the relief he felt that he could shift house. It was not a relief derived from getting away from an unsatisfactory home: on the contrary, it was a much-loved abode and difficult to leave. The relief to his mind was to know that he still had the energy to shift, since the literal shifting of physical location confirmed for him the capacity to stay open and flexible in his writing. A change of house also symbolised the beginning of a renewal phase as he sensed an increasing movement inward, away from the outer, ego-dominated world. Interestingly, not one of the creative people I spoke with expressed any interest in or concern about superannuation. Their response was typically "I'll work till I die", which reminds me of David Malouf's exquisite novel *An Imaginary Life*, in which the main character, Ovid, says, "What else is death but the refusal any longer to grow and suffer change".[1]

The intense connection creative people feel through their work engages them in a continual quest to grow and suffer change. The thought of superannuation, some idealised life in the future, makes no sense, even if they could afford it! They may well have a material need for some financial security as they get older, but they have little or no need to alter the relationship they have to their work in order to achieve this. Sadly, for many others "death" comes early in the form of refusing to grow and change, since the nature of their work and workplace severs them from any meaningful connection with it.

While not everyone can be a full-time artist, we can nevertheless draw some helpful hints from the lives of creative people to ameliorate the ills of the work experience. The central one is to find something that one can do for its own sake, outside work—some activity or pursuit that affords the opportunity to be involved for and from oneself. This would reflect the yin or feminine quality of not having a specific purpose or goal. This is vastly different from some manic, often hedonistic, activity to ease the pain of alienation such as drinking, drugs or sexual binges. These are tranquillisers, not antidotes—they temporarily dull the pain but they don't treat the wound.

By the time one gets to fifty-five and is facing early retirement, or taking a redundancy package, it can be too late to begin to initiate such activities; if all of one's time has been taken up by work, there will have been no rehearsal of doing things for oneself and for their own sake. The risk therefore is depression and an increasingly paranoid sense about one's financial security. What is really at stake here is the well-being and security of the self but, as is so often the case, it finds its way out via projection onto money. After all, for many people work has meant money, so why would it change in the fifties?

Those who can make the change and begin to embrace a broader sense of self can find retirement a valuable opportunity to blur the lines between work and non-work, between work and play, as they extend their engagement in personally meaningful activities. But this break with the habitual view of oneself often only comes through trying and difficult circumstances such as ill-health or forced redundancy.

The moving account of one man in his early fifties, whom we will call Bruce, highlights the difference between white-collar workers and those engaged in physical work when it comes to early retirement. The latter are far more likely to be forced into retirement by circumstances outside their control than to have the luxury of weighing up their superannuation benefits. Bruce was a third-generation farmer who by his

mid-forties started to realise that he would not be able
to sustain the physical energy needed for farming much
longer, and that the farm, in any case, was not gener-
ating enough income to sustain him and his family. In
acknowledging this, he was not just facing a loss of job,
he was facing a loss of lifestyle, a loss of history, and a
loss of a vital part of himself. His wife sought work elsewhere in order to supplement the family income, and
gradually the marriage drifted, finally breaking up. This
led inevitably to the farm being sold up. Understand-
ably, Bruce was left feeling seriously depressed, and the
following four years were very much the dark night of
the soul for him. He moved to the city, where he was
terribly lonely, took an unskilled job in order to keep
body and soul together, and struggled against suicidal
wishes. Somewhere throughout all this, he held on to a
spark of interest in writing, and a woman friend encouraged him to pursue this interest. Around the same
period he had a very short dream, as follows:

> I was back on the farm showing visitors of some sort
> around. There were in the dream three paddocks all of
> which were valueless because the crops had failed. One
> of the visitors pointed out a weed growing and told me
> that if I cultivated it it would have substantial commer-
> cial value.

Many might see this as some sort of wish-fulfilment
regarding a marijuana crop, but in fact it reveals a

psychological truth, that the growth that awaits us often lies in what we reject about ourselves. This truth is neatly captured in an alchemical verse that Jung quotes in relation to a cornerstone that was rejected by the mason who was building Jung's tower at Bollingen, a stone which Jung insisted on keeping. The verse is from the fourteenth-century alchemist Arnaldus de Villanova and is as follows:

> Here stands the mean uncomely stone,
> 'Tis very cheap in price!
> The more it is despised by fools,
> The more loved by the wise.[2]

As a practical farmer, Bruce had neglected his inner imaginative life. But here, in his dark despair, the inner world of dreams throws up hope—and direction, since one can take the weed to be his previously rejected creativity. The commercial value is not to be taken literally, but rather as symbol of the increase in self-worth and value that will come through the choice to pursue his writing. It is doubtful whether any of this would have happened if outer circumstances and his failing body had not forced him to change. But what was impressive about this man was his capacity to grieve, to accept his sadness and to seek help in exploring and understanding it. In short, he separated, albeit forcibly, from his habitual and old sense of himself and embraced a life of uncertainty without maniacally taking off into the outer world. He allowed his depression to work, to initiate him into the next phase of his life.

To my mind, Bruce provides a startling contrast to another man, David. At the time of the interview, David was in his late fifties and semi-retired. Whilst he professed to have a creative life, it was hard to find any vital signs of it during the interview. On the contrary he eschewed his inner life and appeared to find solace in certitude with dogmatic assertions about ageing and life. It is hard to imagine how creativity can survive when such certitude and dogmatism are present. It was equally difficult to imagine how he could be engaged in any form of mentoring, which would have been age-appropriate for him, when he was so disconnected from his feminine self and had clearly denied his emerging androgyny.

In this sense he displayed typical masculine values, although he believed otherwise. The only obvious moment of feeling in our discussion was when I mentioned that he had just passed the age at which his father had died. He momentarily showed a feeling reaction and then quickly retreated back into the comfort of his dogmatic masculinity, somewhat contemptuously dismissing the matter as some Freudian theory. As we will see later, very often contempt forms part of the manic defence against depression. How different a story and how different an orientation these two men exhibit. One through severe depression was able to reflect upon himself; the other refused to enter that world and instead adopted a typically rigid, somewhat contemptuous masculine posture along with an unwillingness to confront his own ageing process and the certainty of his own death. Presumably David had chosen semi-retirement because full retirement would risk exposing him to his vulnerabilities and the associated feelings that would accompany the loss of status along with the confrontation with age and death. For one man depression and creativity was a salvation and initiation into growth; for the other, "creativity" functioned more as a false self arming him against his inner world.

Too marked a split between work and non-work sets up a difficult barrier to the late fifties transition, since clearly it is one aspect of life that must undergo change. Deferring the issue and denying the loss through an idealised yearning for an after-life following retirement is a less than helpful way of dealing with the change. Creative individuals provide us with the clue to negotiating this rite of passage from work to non-work, which for most of us will be completed by sixty-five. It is to bridge the gap between the two long before the actual retirement or redundancy comes. This requires the usual slow process of mourning, often mourning the loss of cherished goals, the loss of power and status and for some the loss of sustaining relationships. Failure to allow this change to occur can mean that work is the only thing that supplies a sense of identity.

I recall one woman, a 56-year-old divorcee with two adult children. The marriage had broken up when she was in her forties, and had clearly left her with some dreadful feelings about herself as a person and her own worth. A reaction such as this often speaks volumes about how destructive the actual marriage has been. It seemed to me that this woman's sense of self had been extinguished in the years of marriage, so that her professional work was the only source of identity she had. She was not able to connect to her past and resisted any attempt at reflection on age or death, despite a diagnosis of non-malignant cancer the year before. She literally kept herself alive through work and revealed an impoverished and damaged capacity to connect. Eros had been, one fears, annihilated by a very destructive marriage. One was left to fear the consequences of early retirement, redundancy or at-term retirement, since work and non-work were miles apart.

Work can act as an anti-depressant for sad disconnected men, but in this woman's case, it was a life-support system. If she had availed herself of the opportunity of some intense and long-term therapy at the time of the break-up of her marriage, it might have helped her to avoid the rigid structure she now found herself in. The outcome for this woman, now in the grip of Thanatos turned in on the self, may be that when she does stop work, she will stop living. The incompleteness of her mourning, which no doubt had much earlier roots, inhibited her transition into ageing and therefore aborted any sense of renewal. Work sometimes provides this, and sometimes not, it is so dependent on an individual's willingness to reflect and allow for the coexistence of work and non-work. These are variables we can neither legislate nor provide superannuation for.

DOING RATHER THAN BEING

One pattern that unexpectedly emerged through my interviews with people in their fifties was a particular approach to life characterised by unrestrained pragmatism. It seems appropriate to discuss it at this point, since it relates to previous discussions concerning work and the role of incomplete mourning leading to an impairment in symbolic thinking. A predilection for concrete thinking is the hallmark of the sort of pragmatism I am referring to. In discussing this I am not wishing for one moment to create the impression that being pragmatic is in itself pathological, since clearly some people are extremely gifted and able in a practical sense. Rather, what struck me was another face of pragmatism that seemed to have emerged as a defence against feelings, in particular feelings of loss resulting from death or separation. As such it is a barrier to actually making the transition, at least psychologically, into older age.

What characterised these very pragmatic individuals was that unilaterally they all expressed no fear of death and indeed mostly indicated they could see little value in even thinking about it or about getting old. Their motto seemed to be to live for the present, but not in some hedonistic sense—in fact, such pragmatism usually negates pleasure, since it is almost entirely work-focused and spiced with a more than healthy dose of obligation.

Whether by chance or not, the matter-of-fact, no-nonsense individuals I am referring to were predominantly female, yet paradoxically their manner of thinking is what one would usually expect from men. They found comfort in doing rather than being, and in focusing on tasks rather than feelings. Yet my experience of them in the interviews was one of exhaustion, an exhaustion that I believe found its source in denied grief and the difficulty of making a meaningful emotional contact. These people tended to say everything was fine, and they presented a picture of themselves as straightforward, competent, uncomplicated people, yet I was left with a feeling of disconnection and discomfort, along with the emotional exhaustion. The odd part of this is that it is extremely difficult to find anywhere to locate the exhausting experience of being with these people, since it is not overt, but covert, covered up by a mask of competence. People who choose this way of being in the world are almost without exception very capable, but the competence is an outer, factual, concrete one and not an emotional competence. The latter, in my view, has been frozen back in time, usually in response to a profound loss such as a death.

The women in this group had two things in common. First, several of them expressed how loved, even admired, they had felt in growing up, and in particular by their father. Second, as far as I could ascertain most had orthodox Protestant upbringings verging on the more fundamental variety of Christianity, so duty, obligation and purpose were well inculcated. Fifty per cent of them were only children. It would seem that as a result of their father's love they had chosen to identify with masculine values. (As an aside one could assert that this same pattern is true for men, in particular men who have identified strongly with an overtly competent and practical father.) This identification with father explains, at least in part, the valuing of common sense and a practical, non-emotional approach to life, and an active eschewing of the feminine principle of Eros, spontaneity and fantasy. For both men and women in this group, a prime concern in getting old was the need to ensure financial security, either through superannuation, or by developing businesses that would sustain the next generation. Whilst all the women were either menopausal or beginning menopause, without exception they expressed little or no concern or reflection upon this experience. To them it was just another event to get on with. One woman said, "There's no point in crying over spilt milk". I felt she might as well have added "There is no point in crying". I was left to ponder whether these people had simply accepted the loss in an uncomplicated manner or in fact were skipping over it. It was difficult not to arrive at the conclusion that the latter was the more likely, since much of their behaviour and attitudes indicated a denial of inner life.

In my view, age was a serious problem to these excessively pragmatic people, but the anxiety, like all anxieties throughout their lives, was hidden behind purposefulness and tasks. One woman said that she hid from others the fact that she was fifty and that she saw herself as still in her mid-thirties. In passing, without any noticeable feeling, she also mentioned that her mother had died six months prior to her fiftieth birthday. At the time I met her this woman was fifty-one. She had not heard the call of death and endings as an initiation into the next stage, in fact she had used it as a beckoning to return to an earlier one, even if this meant a gross act of self-deception. This kind of pragmatism usually excludes the option of cosmetic surgery that we have seen is the preferred option of many women whose physical attractiveness has been their source of identity. The rigidly pragmatic women tend to regard cosmetic surgery as sheer vanity and a waste of money; instead they choose busyness. But one senses that the fear of invisibility is the same, with just a slightly different lyric; in this case it's a fear not of being sexually invisible but of being invisible as a person of worth.

As the interviews with these women unfolded, it was more the rule than the exception to come across loss and death. One woman, Beth, had been a teacher all her life, was in her late fifties at the time of the interview, had two adult daughters and had been widowed for over twenty years. Her husband, who had been quite a bit older than her, had died early in the marriage, leaving her with two young children to raise entirely on her own. She continued to live in the original marital home until not long before the interview. Like the other women, she described her family life as being very loving, but I was struck by the way she glossed over the death of her husband and similarly a scare with breast cancer shortly after shifting house. She had faced one death and one brush with death, but allowed herself no overt expression of feeling about these significant events. It seemed from her account that when her husband died she literally put her shoulder to the grindstone and with a fierce and admirable sense of determination set about, with the help of her parents, to raise her children. But in that magical way that the psyche can sometimes manifest itself in the material world, she recounted how in both her houses she had been plagued by water flooding problems. One felt the houses were symbolically and literally expressing the flood of tears she had not allowed herself. She described a very stoic life, no relationship with men, and a desperate need to be seen as coping. Such an orientation renders grief unacceptable, since if contacted it would undermine the perception of one's self as coping. But getting old threatens this pattern of a purposeful task-focused life, because of the simple fact that there is a diminution in energy with ageing. It seemed to me unlikely that she—and as we will see, this is true of all pragmatically orientated people—would be able to integrate negative feelings: the alarm signs are already present in her attitude towards the breast cancer. It is as if the body is carrying the anger that cannot be consciously acknowledged at the time of change and transition.

Another of these very competent women demonstrated with even more clarity the capacity of pragmatism to deny anxiety about death. The woman had just turned fifty at the time of the interview and revealed a history involving cervical cancer in her late twenties, a severe life-threatening illness in her thirties and a non-malignant breast cancer in her late forties. She dismissed all of this rather too readily and instead the sole focus of her concern in getting older appeared to be her superannuation scheme. In the session, as with the other pragmatists, it was difficult to feel the pulse of Eros; I felt that in not dealing with the anxiety of loss and near-death, she had killed off life itself, so that her pension became the only symbol of the rite of passage into old age. Her situation emphasises how very difficult it is to really understand and accept periods of loss and have a conscious contact with Thanatos, and how little we are encouraged and given permission to express our grief and anxiety. These women's cervical and breast cancer diagnoses represent attacks on the core of their identity as women, yet they could not allow themselves, nor could presumably anyone else allow them, to shed a tear, to cry and express anger at the experience. In not being able to do this they create a large split in their psyche, a splitting-off of feelings from consciousness, which can mean that the feelings find their way into the body, as instanced by these two women's physical symptoms of cancer. Many illnesses have this psycho-somatic base, where the physical symptoms manifest an interaction between unacknowledged or repressed feelings and the body itself. Thus where and how we get sick can often be a rich symbolic expression of what is being repressed. This understanding is beautifully captured in the words attributed to the nineteenth-century British anatomist Henry Maudsley, who is reputed to have said that "The sorrow that has no vent in tears makes other organs weep".

The folly of the pattern of rigid and uncompromising pragmatism we have been discussing is that the person cannot *not* be pragmatic and the "cannot *not* be" inevitably conveys that the pattern is a defensive one, serving to keep out of consciousness any awareness of other feelings that one might regard as unacceptable. In the main these feelings involve the combination of sad and angry feelings which a good Protestant upbringing is most likely to label as "bad". Sad, bad and mad all get confused together and banished, split off from consciousness and located elsewhere, either in the body in the form of physical symptoms or out into the world, resulting in the rigid determination to cope at all costs. Regrettably, in our society the ability to "cope", despite trauma, is seen as the hallmark of maturity.

Thus these people move without processing their

feelings from one stage of life to the next, but no stage brings with it emotional maturation. The incapacity to process separation means that the heroic journey of the fifties transition, in which one learns to integrate opposites and tolerate ambivalence, is aborted. As heroes, or heroines, they refuse in one sense to leave home, the home of familiarity and parental values. The heroic venture, in whatever setting, is always a passage beyond the known into the unknown. Pragmatists of the type we have been discussing are committed to the known, the concrete factual world, since separating from it would force them into embracing the unknown. It is as if these people, along with prevailing masculine social values, regard grieving as evidence of maladjustment, when in actual fact it is evidence of maturation itself. Unfortunately the splitting-off of such feelings inhibits the mourning process and thereby prevents the working through of separation. It is to this moving beyond separation into the next phase of the heroic journey that we now turn. This is the initiation phase when one is immersed in the unknown and forced to allow Thanatos to do its work in disconnecting us from the previous phase or stage of development. Moving into the next phase, as for all heroic journeys, means that one will inevitably confront a series of monsters.

---

1   David Malouf, *An Imaginary Life*, Picador, Sydney, 1978, p. 136.
2   Quoted in C.G. Jung, *Memories, Dreams, Reflections*, Routledge & Kegan Paul, London, 1963, p. 215.

8

Betwixt and Between:
Liminality and Initiation

When speaking of the empty-nest phase, I focused on several women who had made significant shifts in their identity in moving from a false self towards a true self, from an outer definition to an increasingly inner one. I also referred to the shift towards androgyny that can occur when one enters the fifties. But these psychological shifts do not happen in a simple way, and can only occur when the loss or losses entailed in the preceding stage have been accepted. That is when the desire and pain associated with trying to recover what has been lost, whether that is one's physical youth, attractiveness, sense of power or whatever, has been given up and the loss embraced. This process of accepting loss entails digesting and consciously understanding the inevitability of change and the finality that is associated with it. The early experience of being fifty is contaminated by resistance to the recognition of inevitability and usually a person maintains some measure of omnipotent fantasy that somehow one can still alter things and that ageing is not inevitable.

Conscious realisation is absolutely critical for the purpose of achieving separation from the past. In a pragmatic sense this entails ascertaining the deepest cause, or causes, of one's sense of loss and allowing the images associated with that loss to come into consciousness. In short, we need to find the corpse and identify what has died before we can bury it and move on. For some people, as we have seen, the corpse has been their physical youthfulness, attractiveness and sexuality, for others it was motherhood, whilst power and status have constituted the corpse for some. Others, as we have already discussed, need to bury fantasies of having a permanent relationship, and for some women this includes the hope of having a child. Even more difficult to face and finally accept is the awesome finality of death that becomes apparent with age.

Burial is a necessary rite of passage, and finding the corpse allows for confrontation with what is lost. But as we have also discussed, many people cannot get past the denial phase and therefore cannot engage in the burial or mourning. Hence they hold on to outmoded and inappropriate views of themselves, terrified that if they let go they might fall into a bottomless pit of nothingness. They negate any conscious appreciation of change and pretend it really is not happening. Alternatively they acknowledge it only superficially with intellectual platitudes, resulting in the corpse being hidden rather than buried. We all know how smelly and rotten hidden corpses can become! Sooner or later, that which is being denied will reappear, probably in an even more unacceptable form, such as serious physical or mental deterioration.

The function of burial is to enable acceptance of loss and the conversion of something completely subjective into an objective outer fact. This shift seems very important in creating the ambience or conditions for successful transition. In the early fifties the horror and dread of being fifty is kept mostly secret, with individuals fantasising that others would not feel like them and that if others knew how they felt, and what they thought, they would be regarded as neurotic. So the experience remains partly hidden from our selves, which aids denial. But when we allow ourselves to identify the corpse—i.e., when we clearly identify what we have lost—then, and only then, can we make it objective to ourselves and mourn it. Grief studies and research have revealed that seeing the body of the dead person is an important part of the adjustment to death itself. Basically it provides an opportunity to confront and see the reality and finality of death. The same would seem to apply to psychological death, hence the basic importance of giving a conscious realisation and form to our losses. Our fantasies of death, and by implication our fantasies of what we have lost by getting into our fifties, are invariably more frightening than the reality itself.

Burials are the public ritual that gives recognition to finality. In burying something or someone, as opposed to covering up, we yield to the inevitable and accept change as part of life. Life then is no longer perceived as only being a series of beginnings, it is understood to be a cycle of beginnings, middles and ends. (T.S. Eliot captures this beautifully in the "Little Gidding" section of *Four Quartets*.) However, this process of corpse identification is a slow one in the psyche and one that can bring on persistent moods of depression, apathy and inertia coupled with periods of bitter disillusion. The ego is basically slow to identify the "body", or "bodies", since the separation anxiety evoked by the anticipated loss initially calls forth the primary defence of denial, resulting in a strong resistance to accepting change. But if this denial can be finally relinquished, in the face of the reality of getting older, the relinquishment brings with it the beginnings of recognition and acceptance of that which we have lost. This process of recognition is a little like a psychological coronial inquiry aimed at identifying the corpse and ascertaining how the death came about, as a necessary prelude to the burial.

In a practical sense the so-called "coronial inquiry" is the experience of reviewing one's life, one's life goals, hopes, fears and failures, which will of course be accompanied by the recollection of memories, some joyful, some painful. This is the inquiry that facilitates and eventually authorises the final step of burial. But the coronial inquiry process takes time and in my view cannot be concluded much before fifty-four years of age. So the first three to four years of being in the fifties are essentially concerned with the first stage of the rite of passage, that is separation, which means dealing with the grief and sadness attached to one's losses.

If this can be undertaken successfully and not warded off by denial, then the very process of working through the grief and accepting separation leads to a crossing of a threshold into the next stage of the rite of passage. This stage is best known as the liminal stage. The word "liminality" is derived from the Latin word *limen*, which means doorway or threshold. The entrance to a church is one such limen, demarcating the threshold space between the secular and the sacred. Liminality is the classic state of betwixt and between— in the psychological sense, it is the state in which a person's sense of identity is in flux, nothing is fixed, and the ego is homeless.

Within the Greek mythological tradition, liminality is Hermes territory. Liminality is characterised by ambiguity and uncertainty, there is no fixed standpoint in liminality and the normally clear boundaries between "I" and "not I" become blurred. This state of liminality is psychologically created whenever the ego is unable to identify any longer with a former self-image, or persona; and hence it becomes clear why this is the state that follows separation, and indeed it cannot occur without separation. When a person enters the transition of the fifties there is an inner call to cross the threshold into the liminal state and bear the burden of being betwixt and between. One is literally betwixt and between youth and old age.

A 56-year-old successful professional man had a
dream on the eve of his fifty-third birthday which
captures some of this process. In passing, I ought to say
that dreams on birthdays and anniversaries of any sort
tend, more often than not, to be very poignant and
significant dreams. Presumably the psyche engages in a
process of both review and preview. This man's dream
captures the theme of separation and immersion into
liminal space. He dreamt that he had a massive coronary
attack and died on the eve of his next birthday, his fifty-
fourth. In the dream he was conscious of watching his
own funeral, which was held in the church of his childhood. He found himself amused and entertained by the
effusive eulogies, everyone speaking of the high esteem
in which he was held in his profession. He was also
aware in the dream that he was invisible and that his
wife, whose attention he tried to catch, could not see
him, nor could any of the congregation.

Next in the dream he found himself wandering
aimlessly in a very sunny place with a most unusual
light, feeling exhilarated by the sense of freedom.
Finally someone spoke to him and told him that he was
his guide, showed him around and then introduced him
to a group of eight to ten people who engaged in a
discussion with a woman of about sixty years of age. The
dreamer recalled that when it came his turn to speak, he
found himself apologising to the woman about something or other. She turned calmly to the dreamer and
said, "We take responsibility for ourselves here, and

there is no point in trying to please me". The dreamer, somewhat taken aback, then went on to tell his history and how he had died of a heart attack on the eve of his fifty-fourth birthday. He told the group that he felt exhausted and how he had never in his life been able to allow himself pleasure without tying it to work in some form or other. He acknowledged to the group that this was his problem, not being able to separate work and pleasure, or recreation. The woman turned to him and told him, "This place is only about pleasure and reward and it is only in the lower form of life on earth that punishment and exhaustion exist". The dreamer started to feel increasingly better and continued in the group to reflect on his life and death, that he now saw had been brought on by being caught in exhaustion. After time in this place he started to feel different and became aware of the fact that ceasing to struggle lay behind his improvement in well-being.

In the dream he came to understand that he needed to stay in this place until he could come to the realisation of what to do next, then he could return to Earth. He also came to realise through his time in this place that time was the essence of the experience and that the secret to life was yielding. He recalled awakening with a start and wondering whether he was actually dead, because the dream had been so vivid and real.

In short, this very rich dream depicts the unconscious awareness of the need at fifty-three to fifty-four to hold a funeral for his old successful persona and to enter a liminal vague space in which he can learn from a wiser feminine aspect of himself. The lesson he was about to learn was that it is possible to live without being driven by the demands of the ego. One could regard this older woman figure as the anima, and also as a symbol of the move towards androgyny that occurs in the fifties. In the dream he also gets a glimpse of the future way to be, that is arrived at by yielding and ceasing the struggle to control. Yielding is also important with respect to grieving, since letting go is the work of mourning, as we yield to the inevitability of the loss itself.

It was a memorable and moving dream for this man, one that set him off on a very different path, relatively free of persona. The space he found himself in has all the hallmarks of a liminal space, a state of in-between, in which the dreamer could be considered to undergo a form of initiation into an aspect of his true self. This can be seen in the moment in the dream when the anima figure informs him to take responsibility for himself and not to please her. The latter behaviour, as we have already discussed, is a strong component of the false self which is geared towards seeking approval. In a man's case it can also be reflective of the underlying presence of the mother image. It is important to note that this death was symbolic, but it was what shifted him to the other side, so to speak. Any separation from a known or fixed identity is, in a sense, a form of death. It is the dual theme of death and rebirth that forms the cornerstone of any initiation ceremony, a ritual that takes place within the confines of liminal space.

As has already been outlined, rites of passage or transitions are marked by three phases: separation, liminality (initiation) and return. We have up until now focused on the separation phase which signifies the detachment of an individual from an earlier fixed point. In most rituals this separation phase denotes the marker between the secular and sacred space. Separation, as we have seen, enables the shift into the next phase, the liminal. Here the state of the individual is ambiguous. In formal initiation rituals the individual is considered invisible; the neophyte, or initiate, is stripped of all preceding sources of identification, including his or her name. A parallel from our own culture is the initiation of novices into religious life, when they are each stripped of their worldly identity and given a new, religious name. That the neophyte in initiation ceremonies is considered invisible links to the fact that in the liminal phase they have no classification, and in many pre-technological societies they are actually considered dead. So as part of their initiation they may be buried or forced to lie motionless. The symbolic death is a necessary prelude to rebirth, since initiation is a form of second birth and the process of gestation and birth are symbolically repeated as part of the ritual. The sacred place in which initiation takes place is often identified with the place of the individual's origin and therefore frequently is symbolised as a womb by such structures as a hole in the ground. Like the gestation process itself, the liminal space in which the death and the rebirth occur is a space which is considered to exist outside of time and place, lodged between all times and all spaces. Psychologically such a space may well be thought of as the unconscious life, which is also outside the normal constraints of time and space and indeed is the very space within which much of the transformation during the fifties takes place, as instanced by the preceding dream.

Such space that is outside the mundane, material world is often seen as sacred space, as opposed to secular. It is in liminal, sacred space that we confront the very otherness of our being, since in this space the ego is missing or markedly diminished, having been stripped of its solidity as part of the preparation for initiation. To be in liminal space is to be in flux and uncertainty: it is the psychic place in which the neophyte is divested of previous habits of thought, feeling, perception and action. The experience of separation, and the identification of psychological corpses, serves to break the ideas and sentiments about ourselves into component parts and open them up for examination. Victor Turner, the anthropologist who has contributed so valuably to our understanding of the process of initiation, identifies three processes involved in the liminal state, all of which centre around the acquisition of sacred knowledge. The first is the reduction of culture into recognised components; the second is their recombination in fantastic or monstrous patterns and shapes; and the third is their recombination in ways that make sense with regard to the new state and status that the neophyte will enter.[2] He goes on to suggest "that liminality itself may be partly described as a state of reflection" and that the recombination of components into monstrous form in masks and effigies is a means of focusing attention, so that certain matters can be thought about and reflected upon.

If we return to the fifties transition, we can now immediately appreciate the relevance of these basic initiation patterns that anthropologists have described. We have already witnessed how several people reaching their fifties describe themselves as if they were invisible, a theme that was also clearly repeated in the dream we have just discussed. Whilst they were sometimes specifically referring to the loss of sexual attractiveness, it is a discernment that extends beyond this and a sense of invisibility forms a regular part of the experience of being in one's fifties. For men it is often the alarming experience of being overlooked in the decision-making process and the anxious feeling of literally being invisible due to a perceived loss of power and influence. We have also discussed how some women change their names at or around fifty; there may be some overt reason like divorce, but the change is also an expression of initiation into a renewed sense of self. One woman, you may recall, changed her Christian name as a result of a trip to her country of origin. This is a direct parallel to the sacred nature of liminal space and its links to the place of a person's origins, which is why symbols of the womb are often present in initiation rituals. The change of name symbolises a form of rebirth and the death of the former self. Earlier we discussed menopause in terms of it also being an opportunity for rebirth or initiation of a woman into her true sense of self. There are enough parallels to suggest that being in one's fifties is clearly a rite of passage, and if a person can work through the loss entailed in the separation process, then at fifty-four or thereabouts he/she will enter a different phase of the experience, cross a new threshold into the phase in which initiation can occur.

A further aspect of liminality and initiation that we have not mentioned is that it removes a person from the outer world. In modern psychological terms one could see this as representing a shift from an outer perspective to an inner one. In my view this is a shift that occurs naturally with ageing, a sort of acceleration in reflection, musing and recollection. Being in liminal space, around fifty-four through to fifty-eight, is in complete accordance with a natural process so long as it has not been aborted by an inability to let go of the past. What's critical in entering this liminal space is that it is the environment within which the reflective instinct is evoked.

It was Jung who developed this idea of a reflective instinct. He articulated the thought that from a psychological viewpoint there existed five main groups of instinctive factors. They are hunger, sex, activity, creativity and reflection. In discussing the reflective instinct he states:

Through the reflective instinct the stimulus is more or less wholly transformed into a psychic content, that is, it becomes an experience; a natural process is transformed into a conscious content.³

What Jung is saying here is that reflection shifts matters from the physical plane, or world, to the psychological or mental. "Reflection" comes from the Latin *reflexio*, meaning bending back. Reflection is a holding up and looking at, a turning inwards, a bending back on ourselves, a shift from outer, corporeal, instinctive action to internal representation of the issue at hand.

Earlier I said that incomplete mourning impaired one's capacity to think symbolically. It follows that incomplete mourning, the refusal to let go, would also lead to an impairment of the reflective instinct that Jung speaks of. Simply put, incomplete mourning keeps things literal, concrete, out there, on the physical plane and not internal, and therefore not available for reflection. This means one is unduly determined by the outer material world and by the false self. Donald Winnicott, whom I have quoted before, asserts "Where there is a high degree of split between the True Self and the False Self which hides the True Self, there is found a poor capacity for using symbols, and a poverty of cultural living".⁴ Incomplete mourning, refusing to let go and to grieve, probably contributes to the maintenance of a false self which in turn inhibits imaginative and creative life.

The reflective instinct is the mechanism for the transformation from outer to inner, of the literal and concrete into the symbolic. In the liminal stage, according to Victor Turner, previously fixed and given ideas about ourselves that we have dismembered as part of separating are reassembled in fantastic or monstrous patterns. The very monstrosity of these images evokes reflection upon them. Incapacity to reflect on the monsters leads to them being projected out, whereupon one finds one's nemesis outside oneself rather than inside.

So, somewhere in the liminal space of the mid-fifties we will be challenged to reflect upon our own monsters. The obvious question is "What monsters?" And the answer is hidden, distorted fantasies and feelings that are released as a consequence of moving through and acknowledging the separation phase. These monstrous, misshapen, frightening feelings are in psychological terms repressed feelings. Separation seems to have the effect of releasing or unanchoring them from the unconscious, and in the flux and ambiguity of liminality it is as if they float into awareness. In psychoanalysis this process is referred to as the return of the repressed, and it is a process that usually generates considerable anxiety.

In a way it is like a descent into Tartarus, where Thanatos himself resides. Some scribes have the monstrous and misshapen offspring of Gaia and Ouranus living in Tartarus also. These monsters include the Titans, Cyclopes and the Centimanes, who had a hundred invisible arms and fifty heads springing from their shoulders. The Cyclopes, which include Brontes (Thunder), Steropes (Lightening) and Arges (Thunderbolt), are all considered to symbolise the tumultuous forces of nature that lie deep in the underworld of the psyche, well out of sight of consciousness. Turbulence, thunderstorms and disturbing moods often accompany the rising to consciousness of monstrous feelings that we have previously repressed. So when the various losses of the fifties are acknowledged—that is, the loss of youth, loss of meaningful work, loss of children, etc.—the monsters arrive.

Thus acknowledgment of loss of youth evokes monstrous thoughts of misshapen, distorted, weak and sick bodies. Women fantasise that a natural increase in body weight will result in grossly fat, ugly and completely revolting monstrous bodies. Potential or real loss of work can create the monsters of abject poverty, living in the gutter, a hand-to-mouth existence, life on the scrap heap, reduction to a worthless piece of human scum. The loss of the feminine, in the physical sense of menopause and associated hormonal changes, can lead to monstrous fantasies of becoming rampantly masculine, deep-voiced and muscle-bound, accompanied by fantasies of being a dominant powerful figure that would put the average Amazon to shame. The loss of the masculine energy in a man conjures up monstrous fantasies of frailty, vulnerability, passivity, the worst being images of reduction to "an old woman" totally without status or power. Finally, old age and the loss of life conjures up such monstrous fantasies as nursing homes, dribbling, incontinence, totally demeaning dependence and a long, slow, painful death via disabling diseases.

At the liminal point of the transition, use of the reflective instinct becomes critical, since it helps us to think about the meaning of these various fantasies, as the necessary development cannot occur without reflection. Ageing without reflection will inevitably become distressing, seeming to be inflicted on us from outside, rather than being seen as an adult developmental process that we can meaningfully engage with. Basically the failure to turn projection into reflection is a crucial psychological error. It is a failure to move from literalism, an outer-dominated and concrete mode of thinking so characteristic of the pragmatist that we have discussed, to a symbolic or truly psychological attitude. The failure means that a person is stuck with the horror of taking the monstrous fantasies to be literally true rather than symbolic. Without reflection, the necessary initiation into late adulthood cannot occur and fixation at an earlier stage of development is the inevitable outcome. Once again death is experienced as a thief, as a negation of life, and not as a developmental goal towards which we move as part of life. For people who cannot make the crucial move, the monsters are not faced and ultimately integrated, but are experienced as attacking the inner sense of goodness and worth. The result is hopelessness, despair and disillusion. Reflection makes possible, and indeed enriches, the opportunity for bridge-building between outer and inner, between false and true self. Without the bridge a gap exists, a perilous gap or chasm between subject and object, inner and outer, a gap into which we can so readily fall with despair. According to Erik Erikson this despair is

> the despair of the knowledge that a limited life is coming to a conclusion; and also the (often quite petty) disgust over feeling finished, passed by, and increasingly helpless.[5]

Initiation that is undertaken in the fifties and experienced in full in the liminal period could be simply put as an initiation into integrity, since the basic task is to integrate opposites. The first glimpse we get of those opposites is often in a monstrous form. More often than not these opposite feelings have been kept in the dark, so to speak, repressed into the darkness of the unconscious and like anything kept in the dark, out of the light of the sun, it has become stunted and distorted. Thus our first glimpse of these other aspects of ourselves often prompts horror and dismay and an impulse to return to the material world, some place outside ourselves, where we feel temporarily safer. It seems to me that reflection and the reflective process is forever under siege from projection, that is, the urge to place these feelings outside ourselves. The desire to be connected to the inner is always threatened by an equally compelling desire to return the matters, or the monsters, to the outer world and disconnect from them, thereby passing up an opportunity for self-development.

In some ways we could consider the fate of Narcissus, in the ancient Greek myth, not to be so much that he fell in love with his own reflection and died, but rather that he could not stick with the reflection, could not internalise what he saw and instead continued to externalise and project his image onto the physical plane. As a consequence he fell in love with the literal image rather than the symbolic one. Indeed the poet Ovid in *Metamorphoses* describes Narcissus when he comes across his own image in the water:

> I am he, I know; my image
> doesn't trick me: I burn with love of myself:
> I stir my own fire! what shall I do?
> Ask for something? be asked? ask what?[6]

In his bewilderment Narcissus falls into despair and hopelessness and ultimately death, since he is unable to utilise the reflection. This would apply equally well today to many people reaching their mid-fifties. In particular it applies to so-called narcissistic people who seek confirmation of their identity outside themselves, whether that be in the form of a greedy materialism, self-aggrandisement, or in cosmetic surgery aimed at beautification. All of these are outer solutions to inner issues, they are projective solutions rather than reflective ones.

But how do we face the monsters? What does it mean to reflect on them, and what is the meaning of an initiation into integrity? These questions form the basis of the next section which will finally lead us to the third stage of this rite of passage, the return.

MYTHOLOGY AS A GUIDE TO THE RITE OF PASSAGE

There exist a couple of models, or paradigms, for this second part of the journey, one ancient, the other contemporary, but central to both is the confrontation of opposites. These include all those opposites we have already discussed, such as youth versus age, dependence versus independence, masculine versus feminine, non-creativity versus creativity, and others. But the fundamental opposition being faced in the fifties is life versus death, whereas at mid-life the predominant opposition is that of masculine versus feminine.

Two models we can draw upon for reflection on this initiation into integrity are both, in my view, mythologies. The first is that of the ancient Greeks and the second is the contemporary one of psychoanalysis, specifically the views of Melanie Klein. I do not use the word "mythology" in any pejorative, denigrating sense.

On the contrary, I regard a mythology as a narrative account that articulates the universal plots that underlie our lives as human beings. Mythic imagination and mythic stories act like conduits, or intermediaries, between the unconscious and conscious cognition. Myths are a vehicle for expressing a reality that we cannot know directly. It is image and imagination that provides for this knowing and the possibility of reflection. In this sense, myth is an indispensable phenomenon that negotiates the territories between factually obsessed dogmatism on the one hand and a form of distressing chaotic void on the other.

They are stories that give imaginative form to the various struggles, conflicts and vicissitudes that beset us as human beings over time. Mythology is the logic of the plot, the form of the plot, and psychoanalysis is in my view a rich and complex contemporary myth that continues to be of immeasurable value in aiding reflection on our lives and helping us to express and give form to a reality that we cannot know directly. In short, it deals with the unconscious plots of our lives. To treat psychoanalysis as if literally true, as some Jungians, Freudians and Kleinians are apt to do, is to defile it with the very literalism and concreteness that it is attempting to transcend.

It was Freud himself, the father of psychoanalysis, who asserted that his theories themselves were a mythology, in a letter to Albert Einstein on "Why War?" He wrote,

> It may perhaps seem to you as though our theories are a kind of mythology and, in the present case, not even an agreeable one. But does not every science come in the end to a kind of mythology like this? Cannot the same be said to-day of your own physics?[7]

So in referring to both ancient and contemporary mythological perspectives as sources for assisting reflection on the monsters that we confront in liminal space, I am choosing to emphasise the value of these comprehensive stories in narrating the significant plots of human life that we cannot directly know.

Whilst this is certainly not the place to engage in an extensive discussion of Greek mythology, in particular the heroic myths, a brief excursion may assist in exploring this question of the monsters of repressed feeling. Consistent throughout all heroic myths is the theme of the hero crossing a threshold and having to undertake the challenge and task of facing some form of monster, typically a dragon-type figure. Of all the stories, perhaps that of the great hero Heracles is best known. Almost from birth Heracles faced monsters. The jealous Hera sent two snakes into his crib, and it is told that he strangled them to death with his infant hands. As an adult, and as a result of a state of madness placed upon him by Hera, he killed his wife and three children and, as reparation, was advised by the Delphic Oracle to undertake twelve years of servitude under King Eurystheus. These twelve years of servitude

we know as the twelve labours of Heracles. Many of
these labours consist of encounters with monstrous
animals, such as the Nemean lion, the multi-headed
Hydra, and a wild boar. Psychologically, wild animals
are symbolic of the instinctual and unconscious forces
that the ego has to confront as part of the work which
Jung termed individuation. The various monsters
found beyond the threshold of consciousness symbolise opposite or repressed feelings that have to be
confronted as part of the process of redeeming them
to the conscious level. Another of Heracles' labours
highlights this point, and that is the fifth labour, in
which he is required to clean the Augean stables. The
dung of the cattle of the King of Elis had not been
cleaned out for years and the task was enormous. This
labour finds its contemporary symbolic expression in
dreams in which toilets are overflowing or blocked, or
the dreamer is exposed in the act of defecation. These
images of filth and waste are striking symbols of
rejected and eliminated feelings that need to be faced.
Heracles' fifth labour is an ancient version of this
perennial theme.

Other Greek heroes such Perseus and Theseus faced
different monsters, symbolising different aspects of
repressed feelings. Perseus has to go to the end of the
world, in itself a liminal space, and slay Medusa, the
female monster with hair of snakes who turned mortals
into stone when they looked upon her. With the help of
the goddess Ariadne, Theseus slays the Minotaur, to

whom annually seven youths and seven maidens of Athens were sacrificed.

We could continue indefinitely with these stories of male heroic actions, but enough has been said to allow for the observation that the dominant manner in which the male hero deals with the monster is to slay it. What this suggests psychologically is that the masculine way of dealing with monstrous feelings is to kill them off, to triumph over them, and to banish them from consciousness.

These strategies contrast with the way in which the feminine heroine or goddess deals with her monstrous feelings, which in the main are composed of profound loss. Demeter, the Greek goddess of Corn, grieves openly as a result of the abduction of her daughter Persephone by Hades and threatens failed crops. Her grief is rewarded, and Persephone is returned for half the year from Hades, thereby making spring and summer possible. In the Egyptian myth of Osiris and Isis, the same theme of profound grief is present, when Isis mourns the murder of her husband Osiris by his brother Seth. She, like Demeter, seeks to recover the lost object. In fact, she manages to do this twice, the second time recovering the dismembered parts of her husband's body with the exception of his penis. The significant theme of both these stories is the willingness and desire of the female mythological figures to recover what is lost, although in both of the stories this does not result in the return to the former state, but rather a modification of that.

I think it is possible to view these contrasting methods of dealing with feelings that have to be faced as symbolising the masculine and feminine principles that we have previously discussed. The masculine principle as portrayed in these mythological stories involves slaying or sometimes capturing monsters. In some cases, capture is the ideal solution, since it often leads to transformation of the monster itself. For example, Heracles is required to capture with his bare hands the triple-headed dog Cerberus who guards the entrance to the underworld, in order to prove that he could do so without weapons. He does this and then returns the monster back to the underworld, also freeing Theseus, who was stuck there. Many women find it difficult to do this, however. Fear often prevents them confronting their own rage and aggression, thereby rendering them unable to assert themselves. In a sense they refuse to wrestle their anger with their bare hands. If we reflect back for a moment on the shift that can occur around fifty from the false to the true self, this is a shift than can require a confrontation with, and acceptance of, one's aggression, if the movement away from the false self seeking approval is to be achieved. Here the masculine manner of wrestling and capturing the opposite seems appropriate.

On the other hand, the feminine figures of Demeter and Isis demonstrate the appropriate manner for dealing with monstrous feelings of loss, a theme that is germane to being in the fifties. They demonstrate how to grieve, and how to collect, or recollect, the feelings back into awareness. Here the action is receptive, not projective, and in each story the outcome of the divine woman's grief is the restoration or continuation of fertility—a symbol for the growth that occurs as a result of adequate and completed mourning. Indeed the solution to these seemingly competing mythological models of dealing with monsters may well lie in seeing them as forming two aspects of the same process. That is, we need to confront and slay our fears of our own aggression and destructive aspects, as part of the initial phase of grief. Demeter certainly demonstrates this face or phase of loss as she threatens aggressively to render the land barren. Then the second phase is to face and confront the sadness, allow for the grief, and following this to recollect and reassemble what we can of the loss as Isis does. That is, we need both the masculine and feminine principles to deal with our monstrous feelings, and one without the other may well lead to further repression, in the case of the masculine without the feminine, or profound hopelessness and despair, in the case of the feminine without the masculine. This idea of opposites leads us into the second mythology: psychoanalysis, specifically the views of Melanie Klein.

Melanie Klein (1882–1960) was a British psycho-analyst whose significant contribution was to extend and develop Freud's original ideas to include the very earliest stages of an infant's existence.[8] She centred her theory around the duality of the inborn drives of love and hate, or what we could broadly term Eros and Thanatos. She posited two early, oral phases of development, called respectively the paranoid-schizoid position and the depressive position. In the first position, which is activated in the early months of life, the infant's anxieties are derived from the perceived threat of external attack and annihilation. In the second position, which begins in the second quarter of the first year according to Klein, the anxiety related to what she terms the depressive position is generated by the infant's awareness of the damage they could do to others with their own aggression and destructiveness. Central to Klein's views is that these two positions are not just transitional phases which an infant passes through and leaves behind, but they are in fact a description of two positions that continue throughout our lives and are activated at any time we experience loss. This is particularly so in the fifties transition, it seems to me, because not only is a person aware of losses such as loss of youth but more importantly of the reality of their own death. Hence the depressive position is evoked. How well we reconcile ourselves to loss is in part, like all aspects of psychic life, dependent on earlier experiences, including early infancy.

According to Kleinian mythology, our psychic life is essentially bound up with the tensions between two contradictory forces, the life force and the death force. Resolution of this internal warfare through the holding of opposites constitutes the development of maturity, in a process Klein calls reparation, leading to an enhanced capacity to accept reality. Because Klein is so preoccupied with life and death instincts, her mythology lends itself well to an exploration of the experience of liminal space. Indeed, one might well say that the depressive position she referred to is in fact an experience that occurs in liminal space. This is simply because the depressive position involves the realisation that Thanatos, or the death instinct, is inside us not outside. Prior to this, according to Klein, we split Thanatos off from consciousness and locate the destructive forces outside ourselves in order to protect the good feelings and aspects of our inner life. This is a pattern she first sees as occurring in the early months of life and she calls it the paranoid-schizoid position. But in the depressive position we become aware of the existence of these forces within ourselves and as a result we experience anxiety. The anxiety is a reaction to the fear that the destructive urges emanating from the death instinct—that is, hate, aggression, envy, etc.—will not only result in damage to others, but may also damage the good feelings of hope, spontaneity, love that we have in relation to ourselves.

When we enter the liminal phase of being in the fifties, with the awareness of death, we reawaken the depressive position and the anxieties that are associated with it. These then become the anxieties that are symbolised by mythological monsters—the fear and anxiety of the damage and destructiveness we can wreak both against ourselves and others, should the monsters get the upper hand. The anger and guilt of grief can also turn in on the self and, if accompanied by intense envy towards others, can impair our capacity to accept and be ourselves. The "if only" monstrous, multi-headed Hydra of grief can emerge. "If only I had made this choice", or "If only I hadn't", "If only I had married someone else", or "If only I had not done this or that to myself" . . . regrets, guilt and self-recrimination can attack and destroy one's sense of goodness and worth. At these moments the death instinct is in command and we can literally ravage ourselves.

An awareness of these negative feelings in the depressive position, and the working through them by attending to the loss, is as critical to the process of adult development, as it is to an infant's development. This is simply because the satisfactory working through of these anxieties leads to an enhancement in the capacity to tolerate opposites and ambiguity, and finally to the recognition that we are responsible for much of our own chaos. Melanie Klein terms this successful working through "reparation", and it results in awareness not only of the existence of opposites, but also in awareness of the struggle to keep love alive and viable despite the presence of the death force. It is in this work that the reflective instinct is of vital importance.

One cannot hold opposite feelings in consciousness unless the capacity to identify, name and reflect upon them exists along with the ability to recognise that they exist within us. All these steps demand the process of reflection and are aborted by the use of such defence mechanisms as denial, projection and splitting. Reflection enables the internalisation and symbolisation of the struggle, projection drives it out and away. It is the holding together of opposites and not the splitting of them, along with the tolerance of ambivalence, that forms the basis of creativity, since the holding inhibits the move towards concreteness and literality. But the task is a difficult one as we have seen so often, the task of bearing the grief and sadness evoked by loss and allowing ourselves to know and name the love we had for those things that are lost. The daring to name the losses and the giving of them clear images in our mind assists the acceptance of reality and the renunciation of our omnipotence and need for control. Eliot Jacques, author of one of the most significant articles on the theme of mid-life and the depressive position, says that working through the anxieties of the depressive position, anxieties that are derived from loss and ambivalence, ends in a position of being "resigned but not defeated".[9] This is very similar to the famous Donald Winnicott phrase "good enough". The acceptance of one's inevitable short-comings and limitations eases the drive towards perfection and also eases the persecutory and tormenting thoughts that can create the feeling that life isn't fair.

However, like all things in the psyche this achieve-ment of a "good enough", non-persecutory and non-self-attacking position is not straightforward, and certain factors can come into play to prevent the achievement of this sense of integrity and acceptance. These fall under the general heading of what Melanie Klein terms manic defences against depressive anxiety.[10] They are very significant defences in the transition of the fifties, since they defend against the awareness of the symbolic world so critical in the working through of the mourning process. These mental mechanisms of defence prevent the initiation into integrity, integrity that is not forged out of some moral precepts, but out of the capacity to tolerate uncertainty, ambiguity and the acceptance of the co-existence of opposites, in particular life and death.

One could consider the manic defences to which Klein refers as being mechanisms, or strategies, for dealing with the monsters of Greek mythology, or over-coming dragons. So they are designed to slay rather than capture and reflect upon the monsters of destruction: guilt, sadness, vulnerability, dependence and ultimately death itself. The defences against these monsters are characterised by a triad of feelings which include control, triumph and contempt. These feelings are geared to prevent an individual from having to recognise how much they valued what is now lost, or potentially lost, and also to protect them from feelings of guilt and remorse. So in the fifties such defensive strategies will be aimed at denying how sad we feel about the loss of youth, or the devaluing of how important our work might be as we are about to be made redundant or retire. Alternatively, under the influence of these defences, we might respond to an empty-nest phase by denying how important our children were to us, or deny that the loss of our physical attractiveness is distressing.

The triad of feelings composing the manic defence achieves this, for example, by behaving in a controlling manner that appears to obviate the need for dependence on others. It is clearly the defence that comes into operation for those individuals who have denied their own dependency needs. These are the people we have spoken of earlier, who through some traumatic childhood experience, decided to avoid any situations in which they would ever have to rely on others again. As they move into their fifties the misshapen monster arrives in the image of a complete and utter demeaning dependence on others, and this image evokes the manic defence of control. This can take the form of obsessively worrying about one's future finances or job security and even determining to keep working well beyond retirement years. This choice to continue work is made not so much on the basis of satisfaction, as to avoid any possibility of having to rely on others. It is this very thought of relying on others that evokes the dread, or monster, of abandonment, and that in turn calls forth the defence of control. The fantasy lying embedded in this defence mechanism is that if you can control everything, then you will not have to depend on anyone else. But of course the increasing frailty of the ageing body must inevitably be a continuing source of anxiety, and hence this defence is destined to finally break down.

The manic-defensive feeling of triumphing over is aimed at proving to oneself that one can overcome the feelings connected with loss. The workaholic individual is a prime example. The thing about workaholics is that they cannot *not* work, and if they do, then the triumphing over uncertainty and other feelings threatens to break down and profound loss pours through the gaps. Such triumphant people, more often men than women, are also very much inclined to scoff at expressions of concern, loss and grief at getting older. "You're only as old as you feel" is often the triumphant battle-cry of the person driven by a manic defence. The obsessive pragmatists that we spoke of in an earlier section are another example of the utilisation of control and triumph. They avoid any contact with the inner world through their monocular focus on the outer world and action. Reflection for them will inevitably wither on the vine of triumphant and controlling action.

Both controlling and triumphing behaviour can also be seen in marriages where one or both partners will keep their focus firmly on the outside and refuse to either share or reflect upon the grief and anxiety about one of them dying. One controlling partner can exert a strong embargo upon the other of discussing such feelings related to loss . . . "Don't be such a wet blanket" or "Don't be so morbid" are the retorts of the triumphantly defensive partner to any request by the other to share feelings about getting old and dying.

It follows naturally that the third type of the manic

defence, contempt, will be intertwined with both control and triumphing, in meeting the goal of slaying one's monsters. Contempt functions as a defence by devaluing those aspects or things in life that threaten to awaken loss and evoke mourning. So young people are treated contemptuously by some fifty-year-old individuals, as a means of warding off their own grief and anger at losing their youth. "What would you know about it?" can be the typical attitude of a defensive 55-year-old-plus to their children or younger colleagues. Envy is built into this defensive behaviour and, like contempt, it is unconsciously aimed at devaluing the envied thing or person, as a way of denying its real significance. So one can hear the envious person saying such things as "Well, that's not much good anyway" as an expression of their underlying envy.

The overall effect of the manic defence mechanism that we have been discussing is to deny the existence of a psychic reality or inner world. Whether it be by control, triumph or contempt, either singly or together, the effect and the intent is to obliterate any awareness of an inner life. The net effect of the denial of psychic reality is, as we have so often discussed, the impairment of symbolic thought and imagination and consequently the inhibition of mourning. The end result of this is a fixation in the outer, literal, material world. This very fixation can at times manifest itself in a form of rigid dogmatism which is often fraudulently passed off as factual knowledge. But if we cannot allow for an inner reality it is nigh impossible to allow for ambiguity and the coexistence of opposites within us. Thus rigidity and dogmatism which can appear with regularity in older people, will sometimes find its way out in religious or other ideological avenues. Hence we can witness people asserting with complete authority that they know and have the truth, whether it be about God, politics, or the New Age phenomenon. But behind this certitude, manifested in "isms", is a refusal to be initiated and to endure the critical middle phase of uncertainty that exists as part of any rite of passage. It is surely a relief to know with certitude, but it is also an illusion, since lying behind the certitude is the unknown of death itself.

DEATH AND LIMINALITY

Death, the greatest unknown of all, comes into awareness as we enter the fifties. If liminality exposes us to opposites, sometimes in monstrous form, then death is the largest monster, since it threatens us with the demise of life itself. This can provoke a defensive response—some people of fifty-plus may find themselves charging maniacally into new ventures, driven by the thought that time is running out. Trying to control, triumph over, or contemptuously dismiss one's death is at best foolhardy. It requires the slower process of restoring and maintaining a connection to life in the face of the inevitability of death. Whilst manic behaviour can temporarily forestall anxiety and give an illusory feeling of renewal, it must, in the long run, then give way to an acceptance of the reality of one's death if maturation is to occur. This acceptance, which comes in the mid-fifties, can facilitate a genuine renewal of life in the face of death, and alongside it.

Through rites, legends and mythological images, humans have struggled from time immemorial to come to terms with the reality and experience of death. The earliest images tend to see death as a demon who mysteriously snatches or steals life away. This is embodied in monstrous figures such as carrion-eating beasts of prey, often wolfhounds or sinister birds. Death then is symbolised as a devouring monster who has to be avoided and escaped from, or triumphed over and eliminated altogether. In the Greek mythological tradition, Cerberus the triple-headed dog is a symbol of death. He guards the entrance to the Underworld, and as we have already seen, Heracles had to wrestle him with bare hands in order to deal with death, as his twelfth and final labour. The gorgon Medusa with her snake hair is another figure of the death demon (snakes, are associated with rebirth but also in many myths with death). The Harpies who reside in Tartarus along with Thanatos are death demons. According to tradition they were winged beasts with vulture bodies and claws at the end of human hands and legs, and they snatched humans away swiftly and suddenly. In the Anglo-Saxon tradition death is associated with the raven, a word that is linked to the German "valkyrie", another death-demon bird. We could go on and on, but suffice to say that among the monsters appearing at the liminal stage the devouring monster of death is most clearly included, and has been for the human species throughout time. But flight or fight are primitive mechanisms for dealing with death, and modern psychoanalytic mythology provides some alternative possibilities, in particular integration of the powerful duality of life and death. The alternative of using denial leaves death and the death instinct, Thanatos, in its monstrous, devouring, life-stealing, terrifying and consequently persecuting form.

As has been said several times in one way or another throughout this book, death—the awareness of one's own death and the experience of people close to us dying—is the great initiator that calls us into the challenge of further psychological development. We have also seen that this awareness of death, in particular one's own, is an inevitable part of the experience of entering the fifties. For some, this awareness is evoked by parents or peers dying; for others by the observation that they are reaching the same age at which their parents had died, or by the experience of a life-threatening illness. Within psychoanalytic mythology one response to the anxiety evoked by the awareness of death is to resort to the manic defences we have just discussed. So workaholism is one typical response to the threat of death, a regression into doing and pragmatism that short-circuits any possibility of reflection. Others might resort to defence mechanisms more characteristic of what Melanie Klein termed the paranoid-schizoid position, such as splitting, where the threat is seen as coming from outside. In splitting death off from consciousness, such people deny that they will die and see it as something that happens to other people, or project it out into the world where it can form phobias. (No one is likely to go around saying this, but at the unconscious level this can be the belief that is operating.) Another defensive expression of the paranoid-schizoid position is idealisation where badness, and in particular one's death and destructive wishes, are completely denied and split off from conscious awareness and the world and self are seen as inherently and exclusively good. This can show up in some individuals choosing to embrace indiscriminately some New Age belief system, or converting to some form of fundamental religion. What these solutions offer is the illusion that one can avoid confronting one's own dark and destructive side, by locating it externally, outside and disconnected from oneself. But what gives these people away is the very inflexibility and obsessive manner with which they embrace their new-found truth, with the implication that if only the rest of us knew the same truth we also would be devoid of doubt and uncertainty. Idealisation is a defence against loss, invariably promising some version of paradise and not earthiness, where good and bad, love and hate intermingle.

The manner in which we face or deny the psychic reality of Thanatos and our own death is, at least from the psychoanalytic perspective, markedly influenced by previous experiences of loss as far back as infancy. According to Klein the earliest experiences of life affect the relative balance of what she would term good and bad objects, which we could rephrase in more general terms as the relative balance of power of the life and the death instinct. As life unfolds, this struggle with the relative balance constitutes what she terms the depressive position, a psychological state that is awakened at any time of substantial change or transition, since change involves loss. At fifty and beyond, the perception of loss is powerful since not only is it shaped by the loss of youth, but now also by the conscious awareness of the loss of life. So how we have managed to deal with previous transitions, in particular mid-life, will once again play a major role in how we deal with the question of death.

So far we have discussed the psychological task we are initiated into at fifty or thereabouts as the integration of opposites—youth and age, dependence and independence, masculine and feminine, creativity and work. In these challenges the task is to hold youthfulness in age, dependence within independence, etc., but in many ways these challenges could be considered to be preliminary bouts to the main one of life and death, since it is this pair of opposites that provide the *raison d'être* for all the others. An obsessive concern with any one of them—for example, the youth–age polarity—can serve to distract and defend a person from the question of death and how to integrate this with life. Yet the same process is involved psychologically, that is how to get the balance, so that the thought of death does not gain the ascendance to such an extent that it obliterates life. Nor must the desire for life, as in idealisation, obliterate the threat of death.

What is of vital importance in enabling integration is the position from which we view death. If one is outer-directed and one's ego is identified with the false self, then death must surely be seen as the most dreadful loss, a catastrophe, an awful final negation of life. These perceptions will be accompanied by profound feelings of sadness, distress and possible engulfment in despair and hopelessness. In such cases it is easy to see why a person would resort to manic defences or idealisation, if only to generate some antidote of hope, albeit illusory. We have already discussed how the false self works against reflection and is often formed out of incomplete mourning, thereby negating an awareness of an inner, non-material life. But working through depressive anxieties via the losses involved in getting older prepares the psyche for holding the primal opposites of life and death in balance. By this rehearsal, people can gain confidence in their capacity to sustain good feeling about their selves, despite the presence of destructive urges. They gradually learn that Eros can withstand Thanatos and live alongside it.

But this holding in balance requires a more or less successful working through of the mourning process.

The processes of letting go and developing a capacity to reflect is stimulated by the experience of loss literally creates self-awareness, and shifts the perspective from the literal to the symbolic or from the tangible to the intangible. Death seen from the perspective of the ego identified with the true self is not a terrifying catastrophic loss but an initiation into yet another realm of unknown. Thus the capacity to tolerate uncertainty and to value not knowing, capacities that emerge from the working through of the depressive position, are sufficient and necessary attitudes for the integration of death. No matter how much we want to fantasise and reason about what death is and what happens to us after death, the brutal and undeniable fact is that we do not know, it is a mystery. Individuals who orient themselves only to the outer world, whether this be by rationality or pragmatism, or some combination of both, find the unknowingness of death almost unbearable. They therefore either deny it completely as in the pragmatist, or they intellectualise or spiritualise it into something knowable. Some people have a view that humans are composed of nothing but atoms and will simply be reabsorbed into the atmosphere in some form or other following death. Whilst this is true with respect to the physical body, it avoids the mystery and the angst of not knowing. It is also a singularly material and concrete view of death, and indeed of life. Others take the uncertainty out of death by claiming to know precisely what death means and where we are going after it. It is possible that some form of reincarnation exists, but a rigid adherence to belief in reincarnation has more to do with defending against uncertainty than it has to do with truth. Surely truth is something we are forever in the process of approaching, rather than something we have. It is a state of being, not a possession. Our death then looms as the great unknown, and somewhere we need to integrate our physical demise, the cessation of who we are, with the task of continuing to live and find meaning. In the fifties this struggle has the potential to plummet some individuals into despair, even if only temporarily. However, if we can protect good feelings and aspects of ourselves from the ravages of the death instinct, then an enabling perspective can be found.

If for the moment we could free our thinking from the notion of self as *some thing*, then it opens up a wider lens through which to see this task of self-awareness and the significance of it for the integration of death with life. It seems more useful to think of the self as a process, not content, and self-awareness as the process of creating the conscious integrative space between opposites. In this sense self is fluid, and one can extend this metaphor to say that the further out we go into the physical world the more solid, fixed and concrete becomes this dimension of the psyche. At the outer level of the ego, we are perhaps somewhere between fixity and fluidity—in fact, one might say that one of the functions of the ego is to fix, that is make conscious, that which is fluid. At the level of the persona, or false self, we have moved much more into fixity, a solidity that leads to concrete rigid thinking and a preoccupation with the tangible mundane world. The shift of axis from ego to self may well be considered the process of preparing for death, since at death, the ego, along with the body and the physical reality of our existence, is eliminated. Hence the more self-awareness we can create, the more adequately prepared we will be to die consciously. The greater the space, that one might call self, that we can create, the greater will be the understanding of opposites, including the primal ones of life and death.

The process of integration expands the self-space, allowing for a fertile intermingling and interaction of opposites without the insistent demands of the ego to literalise and split them. From this position of a conscious integrative space, death is something we see as part of life, not the negation of it. Further, from this position of self, or integrative space, we also acquire, over time, what one might call the long view. And by this I mean that when we view life from the position of the ego, uninfluenced by the self, we see it in a linear fashion, as a straight line, with a clear beginning a middle and an end. Hence life is governed by attachment, is goal-focused, is purposeful, and death is simply seen as the end. From the view of the self, however, life is not a straight line but a circle, a series of intertwining circles, spirals of a helix. It does not then have an end, since each "end" is merely a prelude to a new beginning. The fear of loss diminishes as one knows the truth of this awareness and the difference between yielding to it and giving in. As an aside, one could say that this would appear to be the outcome of initiation ceremonies into mysteries such as the ancient Greek mysteries associated with the goddess Demeter and the god Dionysus. These ceremonies usually involved some process of purification, in this situation bathing in the sea with pigs, since pigs were sacred to Demeter. The pigs were then sacrificed and usually the prospective initiates fasted and abstained from drinking as they made their way in procession from Athens to Eleusis. At some point they drank a special barley drink to break their fast and finally entered into a darkened hall where certain rites were carried out, culminating in the initiate being shown visions of flashes of light. While the nature of these visions was secret—the initiate was forbidden to reveal them—it is generally assumed that they had a bearing on death and the theme of immortality. Clearly the goddess Demeter, as an agricultural goddess, was central to these mysteries, since she symbolised the process of death and renewal. The ceremony usually included the twin themes of all initiation ceremonies, of humiliation and elevation along with purification. The outcome was said to free the initiates from fear because they now had confronted death and life hereafter. In our modern terms we might say that when we can shift, or perhaps more accurately, when we can initiate and continue a shift from ego to self, we also see life in a circle or spiral and not a straight line. The latter ego-based view belongs to the first half of life when we are attached to objects, have ambition and seek success. By the fifties the internal demand is to yield, and the circular perception of life facilitates this yielding process, often manifested in a deepening sense of detachment from the material world. Death is the final expression of this detachment.

Confrontation with the prospect of one's own death involves all these processes. The acceptance of our own death is a humbling experience that initially evokes profound feelings of sadness and grief as we grapple with the fact that who we are will cease to be. This is a difficult thing to mourn, since the mourning has to be done by us for ourselves. The American psychoanalyst Martin Grotjahn, in an inspiring article about his own forthcoming death written following a serious heart attack in his late seventies, speaks clearly and insightfully about this task of mourning for the self. He says:

> I think of all the investment I have made in myself; the analysis, endless training, the continued self analysis, the drive to understand, to give insight, and the wealth of knowledge accumulated in a lifetime. All this I should give up? . . . One doesn't need to be a narcissist to find that unacceptable. To say goodbye to myself and vanish into nothingness? Well, it shall be done. Nobody claimed it would be easy.[11]

But somehow, despite the difficulty, and bearing in mind the need for symbolic process and thinking as part of a successful mourning, one can appreciate that the way out of this seemingly difficult dilemma is that we have to alter and symbolise a contemporary version of ourselves that now includes the prospect of our own demise along with our limitations. This process is the one that Melanie Klein has referred to as reparation, a process fuelled by Eros or love, which entails the capacity to bear guilt and loss without falling into despair. The process of reparation involves the accep- tance of psychic reality and the renunciation of omnipo- tent and magical thinking, along with a diminution in the tendency to split the world, both inner and outer, into good and bad, dark and light. In many respects this is precisely the process that Jung termed the transcendent function. He describes this in the following terms:

> The transcendent function reveals itself as a mode of apprehension mediated by the archetypes and capable of uniting the opposites. By "apprehension" I do not mean simply intellectual understanding, but understanding through experience.[12]

Although Jung certainly does not suggest that the transcendent function means "higher than" or "above" (in fact he clearly makes the point that it does not mean this), there is a tendency for some modern Jungians to take it this way, which increases the possibility of both idealisation and intellectualisation. I prefer the term "reparation" because it seems more pragmatic, more down-to-earth, and it implies acceptance and forgiveness of both ourselves and others. It is also better in conveying the idea that integration of opposites is about the fluid integrative space between, not a safer place above. Clearly the struggle to maintain the psychic space between opposites is an ongoing one, a dynamic inter-action in which we will be engaged until we die—and, for all we know, after that! The self has a deeper under-standing of this process of dying and death, primarily because the self as we have been discussing it is, like Nature, derived from the incorporation of opposites. The closer we get to functioning from self, yet not devoid of ego, since we need ego to be conscious of the self, the more compassionate and tolerant we become, and the more receptive to the inevitability of death. These attributes are the by-product of initiation into integrity, including the integration of life and death, that can occur in one's fifties. The overall outcome in the long run is perhaps succinctly summed up by Jung in a memorial address that he gave in 1927 concerning a friend simply named as "J.S.":

> To many death seems to be a brutal and meaningless end to a short and meaningless existence . . . so it looks, if seen from the surface and from the darkness. But when we penetrate the depths of the soul and when we try to understand its mysterious

life, we shall discern that death is not a meaningless end, the mere vanishing into nothingness—it is an accomplishment, a ripe fruit on the tree of life. Nor is death an abrupt extinction, but a goal that has been unconsciously lived and worked for during half a life.[13]

---

1   T.S. Eliot *Collected Poems 1909–1935*, Faber & Faber, London, 1942, p. 14.

2   V. Turner "Betwixt & Between: The Liminal Period in Rites of Passage" in Louise Carus Mahdi (ed.), *Betwixt and Between: Patterns of Masculine and Feminine Initiation*, Open Court, La Salle, IL. 1987, pp. 4–19.

3   C.G. Jung "Psychological Factors in Human Behaviour" *Collected Works* vol. 8, Routledge & Kegan, Paul, 1960, pp. 114–28.

4   D.W. Winnicott, op.cit., p. 150.

5   Erik Erikson, "Elements of a Psychoanalytic theory of Psychosocial Development" in S.I. Greenspan & G. Pollock (eds) *The Course of Life (Vol. 1): Infancy and Early Childhood*. US Dept of Health and Human Services Washington DC 1981, pp. 45–7.

6   Ovid's *Metamorphoses* (trans.), Charles Boer Spring Publications, Texas, 1989, p. 60.

7   Sigmund Freud, "Why War?", in *Civilisation, Society and Religion*, Penguin Freud Library vol. 12, 1991, p. 358.

8   For a clear exposition of Melanie Klein's theory see: Hannah Segal, *Introduction to the Work of Melanie Klein*, Hogarth Press, London, 1978.

9   Eliot Jacques, "The Mid-Life Crises" in S.J. Greenspan & G.H. Pollock (eds) *The Course of Life: Psychoanalytic Contributions Toward Understanding Personality Development. Vol. III. Adult and the Ageing Process*. National Institute of Mental Health 1980. pp. 1–23.

10   Segal, op.cit.

11   Martin Grotjahn, "Being Sick and Facing Eighty" in Robert A. Nemiroff & Calvin A. Colarusso (eds), *The Race Against Time:*

Psychotherapy and Psychoanalysis in the Second Half of Life, Plenum Press, New York, 1985, p. 297.

12   C.G. Jung "The Archetypes of the Collective Unconscious" in *Collected Works*, vol. 7, Routledge & Kegan Paul, London, 1970, p. 109.

13   C.G. Jung, "Memorial to J.S." *Spring*, 1955, p. 63.

9

The Return: the Late Fifties

So far we have explored the first two phases of the rite of passage through the fifties. We now need to focus on the final phase, which has been traditionally referred to as the return. All forms of initiation, whether in pre-technological societies or in technologically advanced societies, come to a point where the initiate must return to the world. Having acquired sacred knowledge, the initiate must fulfil the roles and obligations that come with his/her new-found identity and status. Explicit in the process of the return is the demand that the initiate serve the community. It is the mythological theme, also reflected in fairy tales, of the hero returning from some unknown land and bringing back to the kingdom the wisdom and knowledge of the other world. One can clearly see this pattern in the heroic figure of Christ, who after his forty days in the desert, during which he has faced his monsters in the form of the temptations of Satan, returns to the world and commences his public life of teaching and healing. In the Irish mythological tradition, the mythical figure King Cormac mac Art returns after his sojourn in the other world, where he has met the god Manannan mac Lir and received a cup that allows him to distinguish between truth and falsehood, which in turn enables him to be a fair and just king for his community. In the Greek tradition, Perseus slays the monstrous female in the figure of the Gorgon and then returns to found the Mycenean dynasty. The process of return is perhaps best summed up by the American mythologist Joseph Campbell in his *The Hero of a Thousand Faces* when he says,

> A hero ventures forth from the common day into a region of supernatural wonder; fabulous forces are there encountered and a decisive victory is won; the hero comes back from this mysterious adventure with the power to bestow boons on his fellow man.[1]

If we put these thoughts of Campbell's into the context of modern psychology, we could say that having endured the process of separation from something, the hero(ine) has then journeyed into his/her own unconscious and there faced the opposites within. Through this liminal experience, the person gains a conscious awareness of these opposites, particularly the primary ones of life and death, and comes back to the everyday world altered by this experience. The burning question then is what is the nature of the "boons" he or she is to bestow upon fellow human beings?

Before we tackle this question, which is critical to the process of the fifties transition, it is important to attend to a few other thoughts. First, the return, like the other two phases, is not an overnight wonder. Indeed, each phase is implicitly present in the other, so that during separation we can experience the uncertainty of liminality and also be preparing ground for the return. At any point in time, one phase is clearly dominant, and around the end of the decade, from about fifty-eight to fifty-nine, the process of return is undertaken. Any attempt to return before this would be an escape, a flight away from a genuine return, because the latter requires firstly the difficult psychological work of initiation involving the facing of the monsters.

This timing of the return around fifty-eight or fifty-nine finds ample support in another symbolic tradition altogether, and that is astrology. Whilst not wishing to profess any competence in the field, I find it intriguing to see how other mythologies, or stories about our human condition so often overlap. The language very often varies but the themes persist, and when one can put aside preconceived prejudices, which are usually forged out of a desire to protect one's own territory, the overlaps in knowledge and understanding become readily apparent. Liz Greene, a Jungian analyst and astrologer, describes what is termed the Saturn Return. This occurs every twenty-nine years, so that fifty-eight is the second Saturn Return. Taking Saturn symbolically and not literally, she says:

The Saturn Return is ultimately a process of death and rebirth, the sloughing of the old mask and the discovery of the real—and often less "perfect"—individual who has been growing all along, hidden beneath the scaffolding of conscious identifications.[2]

These thoughts echo the theme that has been central throughout this book, and that is the movement away from the false self toward the true self. As if she were exactly describing the liminal period, Greene says the year before the fifty-eighth birthday "is often one of gradual breaking down, disintegration, disillusionment, as well as recognition of all that is false, one-sided, dependent, and unrealised within the personality".[3]

Another noted astrologer, Erin Sullivan, speaks more poignantly of the return phase when she says: "consonant with the strong sense of personal maturity fostered by Saturn is a radical break away from what an individual has identified with in relation to self and society".[4] A little further on she states: "The opportunity to explore personal philosophy, experience freedom and expand horizons is at its maximum after the second Saturn Return".[5] Finally she concludes that

the remaining years need not see a meaningless incursion into a world of objects and measured accomplishment. One can be enriched by these years if one creates the time and opportunity to work on issues dear to the spirit.[5]

The return phase provides the outer opportunity for continuance of a movement towards the true self, and with diminution in parental responsibility many individuals can evidence striking development in their late fifties as they pursue paths directed by the true self and not by the demands of accommodating to others. This can take such concrete forms as returning to education, pursuing artistic endeavours, or acquiring any number of new skills. In this way one can observe the self that Liz Greene refers to that has been "hidden beneath the scaffolding" revealing itself, sometimes to the disapproval of those closest to the person. Becoming ourselves will inevitably disturb the homeostatic arrangement we have with those with whom we are intimately involved. If the fear of disapproval should take over at this point, the likelihood is that the true self will once again disappear behind the scaffolding of the false self. Paul Tillich, the existential theologian, wrote a book with the engaging title *The Courage to Be*.[6] He might well have been speaking of the task of revealing the true self. This extremely brief digression into astrology confirms that the late fifties are significant in setting the pattern for the future, a pattern we know from various initiation rituals is one of serving the community, along with meeting one's own developmental needs.

The second area to be focused on before we attend to the question of what constitutes a "boon" in Campbell's phrase is that this process of return, like the other two phases of a rite of passage, is neither straightforward nor guaranteed to occur. Some people can refuse the call, just as they may have refused the call to face the monsters. Mostly refusal is forged out of fear, feelings of worthlessness, thoughts of being past it, of being of no consequence and of having nothing left to offer. Sometimes these thoughts will be tinged with bitterness and envy. What is happening here is that the person has remained in the grips of Thanatos. The force of disconnection has triumphed over connection and reconnection. In Kleinian terms, the depressive anxieties have not been satisfactorily worked through, so that the transition from liminality to return evokes the old perse-cutory thoughts. A consequence of this is the experience of being stuck in liminality, which as we have discussed is the phase during which one's sense of identity is severely diminished, at least at the level of the ego. Being stuck in such uncertainty, without much identity and without a sense of status, serves to create an internal world very vulnerable to self-attack. Being stuck in limi-nality also makes it difficult to sustain faith in one's inherently good attributes and aspects. In these circum-stances it is likely that a primitive defence mechanism, splitting, would be reactivated: this shows up in an ever-increasing sense of injustice and a somewhat nihilistic attitude that there is no point to life—we're only going to die, so why bother? In short, the difficulty of sustaining some form of integration in prolonged liminal space is daunting, and the ego invariably solves the tension of opposites by splitting. Rigid, dogmatic and inflexible attitudes can begin to emerge in response to the stuckness, which only serve to confirm for the younger generation that old people are irrelevant, pedantic and niggardly.

Others do not so much get stuck in liminality as never go there in the first place, and therefore if there is any sort of return process it is fundamentally flawed, if not fraudulent. These are the individuals we mentioned much earlier, the ones who refused the call of separation and consequently experienced an incompletion, or abortion, of the mourning process, resulting in impaired imaginative thought. Hence the process of reflection and the awareness of an inner life does not happen for these individuals who proceed into old age on the same one-dimensional physical, material plane that they have lived on for their entire lives. The affluence and comfort of this plane will vary from person to person, but what does not vary is the one-dimensionality of a singularly physical outer world existence. Going into old age in this way is in many respects merely a deteriorated and decaying version of the goals and lifestyles of one's youth—that is, material goals, status and power still tend to assert their significance. These people, like those stuck in liminality, can become increasingly paranoid and fearful that outer forces will damage and rob them of their material security, which represents their only source of worth and being. To exist only in the outer life, without reflection, is to be poorly prepared for any useful return, and clearly these are not the people who are going to bestow a boon upon their fellow humans, at least not the sort of boon that comes with the process of reparation followed by return. Those who live only in the outer world dominated by a false self offer a single model of activity, the exercise of power, and not the values of wisdom, empathy and compassion.

In discussing this process of return one must recognise that by the late fifties, or in astrological terms at the time of the second Saturn return, one is just commencing the return, a process that connects us back to life in the form of a' rebirth or renewal of self. It is not a complete fixed moment in time, like a return aeroplane trip, it is the beginnings of a process that takes us into old age proper. So what we bring back as gifts from the sojourn in the liminal space of the mid-fifties shows how we will be for the succeeding decade up until our seventies.

In exploring this pattern and the contributions that one can make, it is useful to draw upon an anthropological concept that sets the scene for the return. This is the notion that a coherent culture is by its very nature bicameral, that is to say, it revolves around the secular order and the sacred. The secular aspect includes normative rules and expectations along with defined roles and the prescribed and expected relationships between roles. In short, the secular includes all those rules that make possible our everyday, observable and tangible interactions.

The sacred, on the other hand, is that intangible other dimension, that serves to legitimate the ordinary rules of a secular society. It is upon the sacred that the secular actually depends for its validation, since in the sacred recognition is given that there is an otherness, a non-tangible world in which our everyday life is embedded and from which it derives legitimacy. Many objects, people and places become symbols of the sacred. For example, the act of violating a memorial shrine to fallen soldiers, vandalising a church or burning a flag are invariably described as sacrilegious acts, clearly indicating the sacred quality that the symbols represent. The sacred serves to also remind us of our mythic centre, as the anchor of the self, and the source of our deepest notions of identity as human beings. In many respects the sacred, and the values derived therefrom, are also the source of constraints upon rampant narcissism since they organise notions and values of proper behaviour for us, often by referring to our relationship with God or the gods. In summary, sacred refers to the intangible world and secular to the tangible.

In this way we could consider the inner world as an aspect of the sacred, since it is intangible. Hence the self, which is central to this world and serves to give direction and meaning to our lives, is often equated with the sacred. In traditional societies, the sacred is usually seen as being upheld by the older members of the tribe. The tribal elders are the containers and upholders of sacred knowledge and truth, and are therefore highly valued members. Their role is to give form and substance to the non-material aspects of being, and consequently they often are given special powers and privileges within their own tribe. They are essentially involved, as tribal elders, in matters of justice and in making judgements on violations of the tribal values. This contrasts with our modern Western society where older people are seen as both invisible and irrelevant. What this highlights is that we have lost an awareness and appreciation of the sacred, and we therefore have no basis upon which to value the older members of our tribe. In an utterly secular, materialistic culture, old equals irrelevance. But what if we consider the possibility that the boons that Campbell refers to might have some relevance here, some role to play in the restoration of the bicamerality of our culture?

To answer this question we need to return to the potential gains that emerge from the rite of passage through the fifties. We have already said that the initiation that occurs is an initiation into integrity, where integrity refers to the capacity to contain and hold opposites. The outcome of this integration is an enhanced maturity that facilitates and indeed makes possible our taking into account the position of the other as a separate individual in their own right. So the integration of opposites, the facing and acceptance of our monsters, allows us to let others be who they are without us projecting onto them our own dark shadows and then rushing into rigid value judgements about their worth, or more likely their lack of it. Through adequate mourning of our losses—and there are, as we have seen, many in the fifties—we come to accept our dark and light sides, positive and negative, and this act of self-reparation is the cornerstone of compassion. It is not forged out of some externally imposed institutional religious values, but out of the hearth of confrontation with ourselves.

But none of this occurs without the willingness to let go, to allow Thanatos to disconnect us from one stage, work through the middle of a muddle, and then for Eros to do its work and reconnect us to a renewed or modified sense of self appropriate for the next stage. One thing is central here, and that is the capacity to reflect, to transfer matters from the physical realm to the psychological, to be connected to our capacity to give mental and imaginative form to our feelings, conflicts and desires. This awakening of what Jung termed the reflective instinct is critical to the transmutation of projection into reflection, of the concrete material perspective into the symbolic. This achievement is, in my view, the maintenance and restoration of the sacred, where the sacred refers to the intangible.

Thus the future role of people undergoing the fifties rite of passage is to return with the boon, or gift, of the significance and legitimacy of the inner world, the world of the psyche. From this boon will follow others. Having let go the singular important material world of one's youth, one can play a role in society that legitimates the intangible, the otherness of our existence; a role that might well be referred to as spiritual. Having undergone the initiation into integrity, the person entering late adulthood may well bring the gift of increasing wisdom, wisdom that validates difference, sees value in opposing positions and does not rush into moralistic judgements of others. It is the capacity to uphold, in a one-dimensional society, the value and merits of a multi-dimensional view of reality.

As part of the shift from the false to the true self, a person in his or her late fifties has a significant role to play as mentor and model to the younger members of society. In this role as a tribal elder, or crone, the older person will be available through their sixties to assist the young by influence, and example, as they struggle with their own lack of meaning in an increasingly materialistic world. But we are talking of wisdom and the right to mentor that finds its origin in one's own inner reflection; this is not to be confused with knowledge derived from outer sources. The imposition of knowledge upon younger people is an act of power and dominance, not influence, and reveals that the so-called mentor has not journeyed very far within themselves. Mentoring as I mean it in this context involves the ability to provide an enabling, permissive and accepting space into which the person being mentored can come across themselves and their own knowledge.

But without wishing to be too cynical when one looks around at our Western society's tribal elders, predominantly in the form of political leaders, it is difficult not to feel some despair. Most political leaders have built their position on the basis of a persona, a false self, with the overt pursuit of power the driving force, rather than the desire to influence, which requires a working connection to the inner world. As tribal leaders they lack vision, are often emotionally immature and narcissistic; instead of inspiring youth, they disillusion them, and instead of upholding the sacred, they become high priests of both the secular and the banal. If on the other hand we are looking to universities to provide sources of knowledge and wisdom then we would do well to forget that idea also. Australian universities are but a paltry shadow of their past selves, and academics have tended to submit, either willingly or unwillingly, to the corporate ideology and marketing forces that will sell anything. The end result is a generation of young people who have been cheated out of an education, are satiated with information, and left with a less developed capacity to process abstract ideas, let alone be receptive to imaginative ones. Pushing information under the disguise of education can only cultivate literalism, and a pursuit of conformity, of certitude, and dogmatism. These attributes are the graveyard of creativity. It is in the arena of the arts and music that one will most likely find true leaders, such people as the late Yehudi Menuhin and the Irish Nobel Prize-winning poet Seamus Heaney, or in Australia, writer Elizabeth Jolley and the recently deceased artist Arthur Boyd. These highly creative people lead by example, are inspiring and above all else speak from the true self, not the persona, and hence they display both wisdom and compassion.

But in saying this I do not wish to imply we must all strive to such heights. On the contrary, society is crying out for a range of tribal elders and the task of transiting through the fifties is a critical period for producing them—that is, for producing people who will hold up the mirror to exclusively material values and restate and reaffirm the necessity of an inner reflective life that works at acceptance of one's nature and compassion between fellow human beings. This involves the important task of maintaining a vigorous dialogue between structure and liminality, between outer and inner, between knowing and not knowing. This very position enables wisdom to exist and helps to avoid the pernicious effects of dogmatism and authoritarianism that can so easily creep in with age. To stay engaged in this dialogue also fulfils the vital role of challenging the current domination of excessive factual information, the possession of which is often fraudulently passed off as wisdom. By staying connected to liminality a person can hold up the significance and importance of not knowing, a quality that the poet Keats understood to be critical to the process of creativity. He described this quality as "negative capability". In Keats' words, creativity exists "when man is capable of being in uncertainties, mysteries, doubts, without any irritable reaching after fact and reason".[7]

The fifties is a time to see the world as a constellation of interconnected and dynamic opposites. This perspective in turn needs then to be placed in the long view of life not being a straight line, but an eternal cycle of birth, life and death, a constant flowing of beginnings, middles and ends. The fifties only serves to lead one into the sixties and the sixties into the seventies, with each transition involving another shift into the unknown until we reach the ultimate unknown of death. David Malouf, the esteemed Australian author, captures much of what this book has been about in his novel *An Imaginary Life*:

> What else should our lives be but a continual series of beginnings, of painful settings out in the unknown, pushing off from the edge of consciousness into the mystery of what we have not yet become.[8]

---

1   Joseph Campbell, *Hero of a Thousand Faces*, Bollingen Series XVII, Princeton University Press, 1949, p. 30.

2   Liz Greene, *Relating*, Coventure, London, 1997, pp. 244–5.

3   ibid., p. 242.

4   Erin Sullivan, *Saturn in Transit*, Penguin Arkana Series, Harmondsworth, 1991, pp. 86–7.

5   ibid., p. 87.

6   Paul Tillich *The Courage to Be*, Fontana Library, London, 1962.

7   Robert Gittings (ed.), *Letters of John Keats*, Oxford University Press, Oxford, 1970, p. 43.

8   David Malouf, *An Imaginary Life*, Picador, Sydney, 1978, p. 135.

Index

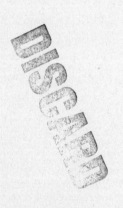